THE ANTI-AGING
DIABETIC DIET AFTER 60

By
Aurora Ross

TABLE OF CONTENTS

Before you start reading, scan this QR Code to get all bonus content!

INTRODUCTION

It might be difficult to navigate the culinary scene and make food choices that are tailored to the nutritional needs of people with diabetes who are over 60. Diabetes is a chronic illness characterized by elevated blood sugar that requires meticulous meal planning to maintain optimal health. Understanding the fundamentals of diabetes and prediabetes is crucial to developing a diet plan that is enjoyable and long-lasting.

The metabolic condition known as diabetes affects the body's ability to produce or use insulin, the hormone that regulates blood sugar. Since diabetes is more likely to develop in later life, it is important to follow a diabetic-friendly diet that promotes stable blood sugar levels. Before a person is diagnosed with diabetes, they may have prediabetes, which is marked by blood sugar levels that are higher than usual but not high enough to be classified as diabetes.

A diabetic diet after the age of 60 needs to carefully balance limiting carbohydrate intake, choosing nutrient-dense meals, and keeping an eye on portion sizes. This culinary journey isn't only about restriction; it's also about finding a range of flavors, textures, and healthful goods that support overall well-being.

The recipes in this collection are geared at the single cook, with a focus on ease of use and adaptability. Every meal is designed with the specific requirements of the chef in mind, providing delicious and healthful options that adhere to the principles of a diabetes-friendly diet. Simply doubling these recipes will allow you to serve more guests or loved ones who may also be struggling with diabetes, as dining is often a social activity.

Explore this culinary adventure and learn about a variety of recipes that not only fulfill the dietary needs of diabetics over 60 but also foster creativity and fun in the kitchen. As we cook and dine together, let's make sure that each meal is a celebration of life and health rather than just something we have to consume.

UNDERSTANDING DIABETES

Understanding diabetes is understanding a complex metabolic disease characterized by elevated blood sugar. Diabetes results from the body producing insufficient insulin or using it inefficiently. For blood sugar, or glucose, to be under control and for cells to be able to absorb and use glucose as fuel, the hormone insulin is necessary.

Here are key aspects to help comprehend diabetes:

1.   Types of Diabetes:

Type 1 Diabetes: Usually detected in infancy or adolescence, Type 1 diabetes is caused by the immune system attacking and killing the insulin-producing beta cells in the pancreas. Insulin therapy is required to treat Type 1 diabetes for the rest of one's life.

Type 1 Diabetes: This form of diabetes is more common and usually manifests in later life. A person with Type 2 diabetes either has insufficient insulin production or develops an intolerance to it. Type 2 diabetes can be brought on by genetics, lifestyle factors, and obesity.

2.   Insulin and Blood Sugar Regulation:

Insulin's Role: Insulin facilitates the uptake of glucose by cells for energy production. When there is insufficient insulin, glucose accumulates in the bloodstream and raises blood sugar levels.

Glucose Production: The liver releases glucose when needed, which aids in blood sugar regulation, such as during physical activity or in between meals.

3.   Symptoms of Diabetes:

- Polyuria: Increased urination
- Polydipsia: Excessive thirst
- Polyphagia: Excessive hunger
- Fatigue: Feeling unusually tired
- Blurred Vision: Vision problems can occur due to changes in fluid levels in the eyes.

4.   Diagnosis and Monitoring:

- Fasting Blood Sugar Test: Determines blood sugar levels following a fast during the night.
- Oral Glucose Tolerance Test (OGTT): This entails fasting and then consuming a sweet solution to determine the body's glucose tolerance.
- Hemoglobin A1c Test: Illustrates the average blood sugar levels throughout the previous two to three months.

5.   Complications of Diabetes:

- Cardiovascular Issues: Heart disease and stroke risk are increased in diabetes.
- Neuropathy: Injury to the nerves that may cause numbness, tingling, or discomfort.
- Retinopathy: Impairment of the blood arteries in the eyes, which may result in visual issues.

- Nephropathy: Possibility for renal failure due to kidney injury.

6. **Prediabetes:**
- Intermediate Stage: Prediabetes is the term for blood sugar levels that are higher than usual but do not yet reach the diabetic range. This suggests that in order to prevent Type 2 diabetes from developing, action must be taken.

7. **Management and Treatment:**
- Lifestyle Modifications: Maintaining a healthy weight, eating well, and exercising frequently are essential for managing diabetes.
- Medications: To control blood sugar levels, doctors may prescribe insulin and oral drugs.
- Monitoring: People who regularly check their blood sugar are better able to make judgments regarding their food, exercise routine, and prescription drugs.

Knowing about diabetes enables people to make decisions about their nutrition, lifestyle, and medical care with knowledge. It encourages preventive steps to avert complications and helps the general well-being of diabetics. To create individualized diabetes treatment plans, people must collaborate closely with healthcare providers.

PREVALENCE AND RISKS

For optimal management, it is essential to comprehend the prevalence and related risks of diabetes among adults 60 years of age and older. In-depth statistical data will be discussed in this part, emphasizing the rising incidence of diabetes among seniors. We'll examine the variables influencing this tendency, such as environmental effects, lifestyle decisions, and genetic susceptibility.

Unique Challenges Faced by Seniors with Diabetes

Managing diabetes presents unique obstacles that call for a customized treatment plan. These issues will be fully identified and discussed in this paragraph. Topics will cover the complexities of managing medications, the impact of concomitant health disorders that are frequent in older persons, and the impact of age-related changes on the body's sensitivity to insulin.

Furthermore, lifestyle problems including altered appetite, reduced mobility, and the risk of social isolation will be discussed. Comprehending these obstacles is essential to formulating efficacious tactics to surmount obstacles to appropriate diabetic care, guaranteeing a comprehensive and encouraging methodology for the elderly.

Impact of Aging on Diabetes Management

Physiological changes brought on by aging may make managing diabetes more difficult. This section will look at how aging affects the body's overall metabolic function, insulin sensitivity, and glucose regulation. It will go through how critical it is to modify diabetes care plans to account for these developments, including dietary, exercise, and medication modifications.

Additionally, the part will discuss how age-related illnesses like arthritis or cognitive decline have shaped diabetes care. This section attempts to arm elders and healthcare providers with information that promotes more efficient, individualized, and long-lasting approaches to diabetes management in later life by offering insights into homaging affect the nuances of diabetes care.

MEDICAL CONSIDERATIONS

Comprehensive Exploration of Medications for Diabetes

In order to attain ideal blood sugar control, managing diabetes in seniors frequently requires a carefully calibrated combination of drugs. This is a thorough examination of the several drugs that are frequently recommended for elderly patients with diabetes:

1. Oral Medications:

Metformin:

- Mechanism of Action: enhances muscle cell insulin sensitivity and lowers the liver's synthesis of glucose.
- Benefits for Seniors: Generally well tolerated, with a minimal chance of hypoglycemia and some advantages for the heart.
- Sulfonylureas (e.g., Glipizide, Gliclazide):
- Mechanism of Action: Increases the amount of insulin released by the pancreas.
- Considerations for Seniors: Danger of hypoglycemia and possible drug interactions, particularly in elderly patients.

2. Injectable Medications:

Insulin:

- Types (e.g., Regular, NPH, Long-acting, Rapid-acting): Distinct insulin formulations that differ in their time to action and onset.
- Benefits for Seniors: Gives exact blood sugar control; in cases of severe diabetes, this may be necessary.

3. Considerations for Seniors:

Individualization of Treatment:

- Rationale: Adjusting prescriptions based on the unique requirements of each senior, taking into account lifestyle, comorbidities, and age.
- Benefits: Reduces the possibility of side effects and increases the efficacy of treatment.

Risk of Hypoglycemia:

- Monitoring: Hypoglycemia should be regularly monitored, particularly in elderly people who may be more vulnerable.
- Adjustments: It could be necessary to modify your medication to lower your risk of low blood sugar.

Polypharmacy:

- Awareness: Recognising possible interactions between prescription drugs for diabetes and other drugs that elderly people could be taking.
- Communication: To properly manage polypharmacy, keep lines of communication open with healthcare providers.

Renal Function:

- Monitoring: Renal function should be regularly assessed because poor kidney function can affect prescription decisions.
- Caution: Dose modifications for medications given to patients with reduced renal function.

Cardiovascular Considerations:

- Benefits: Certain drugs have the potential to improve cardiovascular health, which is particularly important for seniors who are more likely to experience cardiovascular problems.

Patient Education:

- Empowerment: Giving seniors accurate information about their drug emphasizing the adherence, possible adverse effects, and how to take them.
- Encouragement: Encouraging seniors and healthcare professionals to have frank conversations to address worries and inquiries.

In conclusion, careful management of diabetes in the elderly requires a sophisticated grasp of several drug regimens while taking into account each patient's unique health profile and possible obstacles. In order to monitor side effects, and properly customize therapy to enable seniors to take an active role in their diabetes care, regular communication between the senior's healthcare staff and themselves is crucial.

REGULAR MONITORING AND TESTING

Effective diabetes management necessitates routine testing and monitoring.

Importance of Monitoring Blood Glucose Levels:

For seniors in particular, blood glucose monitoring is an essential part of managing diabetes. It aids in making knowledgeable decisions regarding medication, nutrition, and lifestyle choices by offering insightful information about how the body processes glucose. This is why it's so important to monitor:

1. Immediate Feedback: Seniors can maintain healthy blood glucose levels by making quick adjustments based on real-time information obtained from routine monitoring.

2. Prevention of Complications: Regular monitoring aids in the prevention of consequences like neuropathy, cardiovascular problems, and eye problems that are linked to poorly managed diabetes.

3. Treatment Adjustment: Effective diabetes treatment is ensured by monitoring, which enables elders and healthcare professionals to make the required changes to medication, insulin, and lifestyle choices.

4. Enhanced Quality of Life: Seniors can have more energy, a happier mood, and an all-around higher quality of life by keeping their blood glucose levels steady.

Incorporating Routine Testing into Daily Lives:

For elders managing diabetes, periodic blood glucose testing must become a part of everyday life. The following useful advice will help you easily include testing into your everyday schedule:

1. Establish a Schedule:

- Test at designated times, such as right before or right after meals or right before bed.

- As a reminder to test, use everyday activities like brushing your teeth or watching your favorite show.

2. Create a Testing Station:

- Ensure the area is well-lit and comfortable for testing.
- Test supplies should be stored in a designated area.
- Ascertain that the testing space is completely lit.

3. Utilize Reminders:

- Utilise smartphone apps or set alarms to serve as a reminder for testing times.
- Connect testing to other routine tasks, such as taking medication.

4. Keep Supplies Accessible:

- Make sure lancets, alcohol swabs, glucose meters, and test strips are all conveniently located.
- When you are outside the house, think about bringing a portable testing kit.

5. Track Results:

- To keep track of blood glucose measurements, use a smartphone app or a journal.
- Take note of things like food, exercise, and stress levels to get a complete picture.

Use of Glucose Meters:

1. Selecting a Glucose Meter:

- Select a meter that meets your demands, is easy to use, and has a wide display.
- Think of functions like memory storage, voice prompts, and backlighting.

2. Proper Technique:

- Prior to testing, wash your hands to guarantee reliable findings.
- Utilize the meter and lancet in accordance with the manufacturer's recommendations.

3. Regular Maintenance:

- To maintain accuracy, keep the meter clean and inspect it frequently.
- As advised by the manufacturer, swap out the test strips and batteries.

Interpretation of Blood Glucose Readings:

1. Target Ranges:

- Recognize the postprandial and fasting target blood glucose ranges established by healthcare professionals.

2. Interpreting Results:

- Elevated levels could suggest that you need to modify your lifestyle or take your medicine.
- If the reading is low, you might need to act right away to avoid hypoglycemia.

3. Pattern Recognition:

Identify patterns by noting trends in blood glucose levels over time.

Recognize factors influencing fluctuations, such as meals, physical activity, and stress.

ROLE OF HEALTHCARE PROFESSIONALS:

1. Education:
   - Healthcare providers offer advice on the proper usage of glucose meters.
   - Seniors are taught about target ranges and the need to keep blood glucose levels steady.
2. Individualized Plans:
   - Create customized monitoring programs depending on the requirements and lifestyle of senior citizens.
   - Adapt the frequency of monitoring in response to modifications in treatment plans or health conditions.
3. Reviewing Data:
   - In order to make well-informed decisions regarding treatment modifications, healthcare professionals examine and evaluate blood glucose data.
   - Seniors can better comprehend their results and resolve any concerns with regular consultations.
4. Support and Motivation:
   - Encourage seniors to continue their consistent monitoring by providing them with emotional support and inspiration.
   - Acknowledge accomplishments and offer helpful criticism to support constructive behavior.

In conclusion, the key to successful diabetes treatment for elders with diabetes is blood glucose monitoring. Seniors can take proactive measures to maintain appropriate blood glucose levels and improve their general well-being by integrating routine testing into daily life, using glucose meters properly, interpreting data, and working with healthcare specialists. In order to successfully manage diabetes, regular communication with healthcare practitioners guarantees that monitoring measures are in line with personal health objectives.

COLLABORATING WITH HEALTHCARE PROFESSIONALS

Seniors will be better prepared to handle the challenges of diabetes control if they are encouraged to collaborate with healthcare providers. Senior diabetics' general health and well-being are eventually improved by this collaborative approach, which guarantees a more tailored and responsive strategy.

Importance Of Building A Strong Healthcare Team

For people with diabetes, especially those in their later years, to receive comprehensive and efficient care, it is imperative to assemble a robust healthcare team that includes a variety of specialists. The following are the main justifications for why every member of the medical team is essential:

1. Primary Care Physicians (PCPs):

    - Comprehensive Care: As the primary point of contact, PCPs manage the patient's general health. They are in charge of organizing many facets of healthcare and making sure that all illnesses, including diabetes, are properly treated.
    - Preventive Care: Preventive care is the main focus of PCPs, who assist in identifying and addressing possible health problems before they worsen. It's critical to have routine tests and examinations to manage complications associated with diabetes.

2. Endocrinologists:

    - Specialized Diabetes Management: Diabetes and other hormonal problems are the focus of endocrinologists' expertise. Their knowledge is crucial for developing customized diabetes treatment programs, handling challenging situations, and tackling certain endocrine system issues.
    - Advanced Treatment Options: Endocrinologists are knowledgeable about the most recent developments in diabetes care, giving their patients access to cutting-edge therapies and tools that could be helpful for elderly diabetics.

3. Dietitians:

    Nutritional Guidance: When it comes to informing people about the connection between diabetes and food, dietitians are essential. By taking into account variables including age-related changes, concurrent medical conditions, and drug interactions, they can customize meal programs to fit the unique nutritional needs of elders.

    Weight Management: Maintaining a healthy weight is an important part of care for many elderly diabetics. Dietitians can offer advice on how to eat a balanced, diabetes-friendly diet in order to reach and maintain a healthy weight.

4. Diabetes Educators:

    - Empowering Patients: The goal of diabetes education is to enable people to actively manage their illness. To promote independence and self-efficacy, they offer education on self-monitoring, medication adherence, and lifestyle adjustments.

- Continuous Support: Diabetes educators provide people with continuous assistance in navigating the day-to-day obstacles associated with diabetes. They can respond to inquiries, offer assistance with resources, and help solve problems, all of which boost long-term results.

Benefits of a Collaborative Healthcare Team:

1.   Holistic Care: In order to provide holistic treatment that goes beyond simply controlling blood sugar levels, a multidisciplinary team approach guarantees that all facets of a senior's health are taken into account.

2.   Tailored Treatment Plans: The diverse perspectives and experiences of each member of the healthcare team enable the creation of individualized treatment programs that take the patient's lifestyle and general health into account.

3.   Early Intervention: Frequent contact with medical professionals lowers the chance of unfavorable health outcomes by facilitating early detection and intervention for possible issues.

4.   Improved Patient Engagement: Seniors who receive collaborative care are more likely to have a solid patient-provider connection, be actively involved in their healthcare decisions, and follow treatment recommendations.

In conclusion, the establishment of a strong healthcare team guarantees that elderly individuals with diabetes obtain all-encompassing, customized, and harmonious care. This is the only way to successfully treat diabetes over the long term, improve quality of life, and maximize health outcomes.

Roles of Each Team Member And How Their Expertise Contributes To Comprehensive Diabetes Care

1.   Primary Care Physicians (PCPs):

Role: For people with diabetes, CPs are the main point of contact.

Contribution:

- Holistic Assessment: PCPs provide routine examinations, evaluate patients' general health, and spot any possible issues or comorbidities.
- Coordination: They collaborate with other experts to guarantee a well-rounded approach to diabetes care.
- Preventive Care: PCPs place a strong emphasis on preventative care, encouraging regular screenings and good lifestyle choices.

2.   Endocrinologists:

Role: Diabetes and other hormonal problems are the focus of endocrinologists' expertise.

Contribution:

- Specialized Treatment: They offer specialized diabetes care, particularly in situations where following standard control may be difficult.
- Medication Adjustments: Endocrinologists customize drug schedules to meet patient demands and treatment response differences.
- Advanced Interventions: Endocrinologists can recommend sophisticated therapies, such as continuous glucose monitoring or insulin pump therapy, for complicated cases.

3.   Dietitians:

Role: Dietitians concentrate on dietary recommendations and nutritional factors for people with diabetes.

Contribution:

- Nutritional Guidance: They create customized meal plans that take dietary requirements, cultural factors, and particular health conditions into account.
- Education: Dietitians teach people how to maintain their blood sugar levels by controlling portion sizes, monitoring carbohydrates, and making well-informed food choices.
- Weight Management: They offer weight control techniques, which are frequently essential for the management of diabetes.

4. *Diabetes Educators:*

Role: Diabetes educators enable people to self-manage their illness.

Contribution:

- Patient Education: They offer comprehensive instruction in managing diabetes on one's own, covering things like blood glucose monitoring, medication administration, and identifying potential problems.
- Lifestyle Modification: Diabetes educators help people make and maintain dietary, physical activity, and stress-reduction improvements in their lives.
- Behavioral Support: They encourage commitment to treatment plans and provide behavioral techniques for overcoming obstacles.

Benefits of Collaborative Care:

1. Comprehensive Approach: Because each team member brings a unique set of skills to the table, diabetes treatment is provided in a holistic manner that takes behavioral, dietary, and medical factors into account.

2. Personalization: Personalised treatment regimens that take into account each patient's particular needs, preferences, and obstacles are made possible via collaborative care.

3. Timely Interventions: Team members who communicate regularly can identify problems early and take appropriate action to stop diabetes-related complications from getting worse.

4. Patient Empowerment: People are empowered to take an active role in their treatment, make educated decisions, and successfully manage their diabetes on a daily basis because of the healthcare team's collective experience.

In conclusion, a comprehensive and customized approach to diabetes care is made possible by the combined efforts of primary care doctors, endocrinologists, nutritionists, and diabetes educators. This all-encompassing approach raises patient outcomes, increases the efficacy of therapies, and advances the general well-being of those with diabetes.

VARIOUS TRICKS YOU NEED TO WATCH OUT FOR

In order to properly manage blood sugar levels, managing a diabetic diet after the age of 60 necessitates a careful understanding of numerous important elements. The following are some tips and things to remember:

Carbohydrate Management:

- Choose Complex Carbs: Choose veggies that are high in fiber, lentils, and whole grains. The effect on blood sugar levels of these complex carbs is kinder.
- Portion Control: Pay attention to portion sizes to prevent consuming too many carbohydrates, as this might cause blood sugar to increase. To determine the proper serving sizes, use measurement devices or become acquainted with visual cues.

Balanced Plate Approach:

- Include Proteins: Include lean proteins in your diet, such as fish, poultry, tofu, and lentils, to help control blood sugar levels and encourage feelings of fullness.
- Healthy Fats: Include foods high in unsaturated fats, such as avocados, almonds, and olive oil, to promote fullness and delay the breakdown of carbohydrates.

Mindful Eating:

- Eat Slowly: Eat slowly and deeply, enjoying every taste. Eating slowly can facilitate better digestion and portion control.
- Stay Present: Be aware of what you're eating and your body's signals of hunger and fullness. By doing so, overeating can be avoided and a positive relationship with food can be fostered.

Sugar Awareness:

- Read Labels: To identify any hidden sugars, carefully read food labels. Added sugars are included in many processed foods and are also referred to as fructose, sucrose, or high fructose corn syrup.
- Natural Sweeteners: As a moderate substitute for processed sugars, use natural sweeteners like stevia or monk fruit.

Regular Monitoring:

- Blood Sugar Testing: Monitor your blood sugar levels on a regular basis, particularly after eating. This enables you to promptly modify your diet plan and helps you comprehend how various foods affect your body.

Hydration:

- Water Intake: Drink lots of water to stay hydrated. Avoid sugar-filled beverages as they can cause blood sugar levels to rise quickly.

Meal Timing:

- Consistent Schedule: To control blood sugar levels, try to stick to a regular eating routine. Meals should be spread out throughout the day to avoid significant swings.

Physical Activity:

- Regular Exercise: Maintaining a regular exercise schedule can help lower blood sugar and increase insulin sensitivity. To choose a safe exercise program, speak with a healthcare provider.

Personalized Approach:

- Individualized Needs: Understand that each person's body reacts to food in a unique way. Keep an eye on how particular meals affect your blood sugar levels and adjust your diet accordingly.

You can make a diabetic diet that promotes your health and provides a varied and fulfilling culinary experience by implementing these tips and considerations into your daily routine. Recall that treating diabetes and enhancing general well-being can benefit greatly from minor changes.

PRACTICAL TIPS ON HOW TO COPE WITH LIFE WITH DIABETES

Living a healthy lifestyle and using practical tactics are key components of treating diabetes.

Medication Adherence:

- Follow Prescribed Regimen: Adhere to your doctor's prescriptions for medication. Talk to your healthcare practitioner about any worries you may have or any side effects you may be experiencing to determine the best course of action.

Stress Management:

- Relaxation Techniques: Include stress-relieving exercises in your regular routine, such as yoga, meditation, or deep breathing. Blood sugar levels can be impacted by prolonged stress, therefore it's important to learn how to unwind.

Regular Check-ups:

- Healthcare Team Support: Keep up with routine check-ups with your medical team. Frequent evaluations enable you to monitor your development and make any necessary modifications to your diabetes treatment strategy.

Community Support:

- Join Support Groups: Make connections with people who also have diabetes. It can be encouraging and foster a feeling of community to share stories and advice.

Educate Yourself:

- Stay Informed: Find out about managing diabetes. Knowing the illness gives you the power to make wise choices regarding your nutrition, way of life, and general health.

Celebrate Successes:

- Small Achievements Matter: Throughout your diabetes journey, recognize and celebrate your little triumphs. Every action counts, whether it's establishing a new healthy habit or keeping blood sugar levels steady.

Recall that managing diabetes is a journey that calls for small, long-term adjustments. You may take charge of your health and have a happy, active life by implementing these doable suggestions into your everyday routine. For individualized counsel and direction catered to your unique needs, always seek the assistance of your healthcare team.

NUTRITIONAL BASICS FOR DIABETES

A balanced, nutrient-rich diet is more important as people age, especially for those who are managing diabetes.

A well-balanced diet that is abundant in vital nutrients, vitamins, and minerals is critical for the efficient management of diabetes. These elements are essential for maintaining general health, controlling blood sugar levels, and averting problems from diabetes. An outline of their effects is provided below, with a focus on immune system performance, energy levels, and preventing complications:

I. Essential Nutrients and Diabetes:

Proteins:

- Role: Vital for the upkeep and repair of muscles.
- Impact on Diabetes: Maintains steady blood sugar levels, helps control weight, and promotes general physical health.

Carbohydrates:

- Role: The body's main source of energy.
- Impact on Diabetes: In order to control blood sugar levels, it is essential to monitor carbohydrate intake. Pay attention to complex carbs to avoid sudden increases in energy.

Fats:

- Role: Essential for the synthesis of hormones, including insulin.
- Impact on Diabetes: Good fats, such as omega-3 fatty acids, may reduce inflammation and promote cardiovascular health.

Fiber:

- Role: Promotes healthy digestion and aids in blood sugar regulation.
- Impact on Diabetes: Reduces the rate at which glucose is absorbed, helping to improve blood sugar regulation and support weight loss.

VITAMINS AND DIABETES:

Vitamin D:

- Role: Enhances the immune system and bone health.
- Impact on Diabetes: This may contribute to reducing inflammation and increasing insulin sensitivity.

Vitamin C:

- Role: An antioxidant that promotes the healing of wounds and the immune system.
- Impact on Diabetes: Reduces the inflammation and oxidative stress brought on by diabetes.

B Vitamins (B6, B12, Folate):

Role: Important for the production of red blood cells, energy metabolism, and neuronal function.

Impact on Diabetes: Helps with glucose metabolism, promotes nerve function, and may help lower the incidence of diabetic neuropathy.

MINERALS AND DIABETES:

Magnesium:

- Role: Supports blood glucose management, and muscle and neuron function.
- Impact on Diabetes: This could be helpful in improving blood sugar regulation and helping to increase insulin sensitivity.

Chromium:

- Role: Supports the metabolism of glucose and the action of insulin.
- Impact on Diabetes: May increase blood sugar regulation and insulin sensitivity.

Zinc:

- Role: Vital for wound healing and immunological function.
- Impact on Diabetes: Enhances general health and strengthens the immune system.

ENERGY LEVELS AND DIABETES:

Role of Macronutrients:

- Balanced Intake: Guarantees a consistent flow of energy all day long.
- Impact on Diabetes: Helps maintain steady blood sugar levels and reduces swings in energy.

4.2 Hydration:

- Role: Vital for preserving energy levels and promoting general wellness.
- Impact on Diabetes: This keeps you from becoming dehydrated, which can impair your energy and cognitive abilities.

IMMUNE FUNCTION AND DIABETES:

Antioxidants:

- Role: Shield cells from oxidative damage while boosting the immune system.
- Impact on Diabetes: Lowers inflammation and might assist in reducing the consequences of diabetes.

Vitamin D:

- Role: Controls the immunological system.
- Impact on Diabetes: Sufficient amounts could support a healthy immune system.

PREVENTION OF COMPLICATIONS:

Cardiovascular Health:

- Omega-3 Fatty Acids: Encourage heart health and lower your chance of developing diabetes-related cardiovascular problems.

Nerve Health:

- B Vitamins (B6, B12): Lessen the chance of developing diabetic neuropathy by supporting nerve health.

Bone Health:

- Calcium and Vitamin D: Vital to preserve healthy bones, lower the incidence of fractures, and promote general well-being.

In conclusion, vitamins, minerals, and vital nutrients all have a variety of roles in the control of diabetes. They affect immune system performance, and energy levels, and help avoid diabetes-related problems. The key to promoting general health and well-being in people with diabetes is a diet that is nutrient-rich, well-balanced and well-managed. Diabetes sufferers must collaborate with medical professionals to develop individualized nutrition regimens that address their unique requirements.

INCORPORATING NUTRIENT-RICH FOODS INTO DAILY MEALS (PRACTICAL TIPS)

A diet high in nutrients is crucial for seniors, especially those with diabetes. The following useful advice will provide seniors with the knowledge they need to make dietary decisions that support their general health and diabetes management:

1. Prioritize Whole, Unprocessed Foods:

- Choose Whole Grains: Choose whole grains over refined grains, such as quinoa, brown rice, and whole wheat bread.
- Add Some Lean Proteins: Add sources of lean protein such as fish, poultry, beans, and tofu.

2. Embrace Colorful Fruits and Vegetables:

- Varied Colors: In order to guarantee a wide variety of nutrients, aim for a vibrant choice of fruits and vegetables.
- Fresh or Frozen: While frozen vegetables are both nutritious and convenient, fresh produce is still the best choice.

3. Opt for Healthy Fats:

- Choose Omega-3 Rich Foods: Add walnuts, flaxseeds, chia seeds, and fatty fish (salmon, mackerel) to your diet for heart-healthy omega-3 fatty acids.
- Use Healthy Oils: For cooking and dressings, use canola, avocado, or olive oil.

4. Manage Carbohydrates Mindfully:

- Focus on Complex Carbs: Select complex carbs for long-lasting energy and blood sugar regulation, such as whole grains, legumes, and sweet potatoes.
- Watch Portion Sizes: Pay attention to portion proportions to prevent consuming too many carbohydrates.

5. Include High-Fiber Foods:

- Add Fiber-Rich Foods: To promote digestive health, include high-fiber foods such as whole grains, beans, and lentils.
- Snack on Nuts and Seeds: Rich in fiber and good fats are almonds, chia seeds, & flaxseeds.

6. Prioritize Lean Proteins:

- Lean Meat Options: Select protein sources low in saturated fat, such as fish, poultry without skin, and lean meat cuts.
- Plant-Based Proteins: For variation, add plant-based proteins such as tofu, lentils, and beans.

7. Mindful Meal Planning:

- Create Balanced Meals: For long-lasting energy, make sure every meal consists of a combination of healthy fats, proteins, and carbs.

- Plan Snacks: Keep wholesome snacks close at hand to prevent reaching for bad choices.

8. Control Sodium Intake:

- Use Herbs and Spices: Instead of adding too much salt, enhance the flavor with herbs, spices, and lemon.
- Choose Low-Sodium Options: Choose tinned goods, sauces, and condiments with lower salt content.

9. Stay Hydrated:

- Water is Key: Stay hydrated and promote general health throughout the day by drinking lots of water.
- Limit Sugary Drinks: Reduce the amount of sugar-filled drinks you consume and substitute water, herbal teas, or flavored water.

10. Practice Portion Control:

- Use Smaller Plates: To assist you in managing portion sizes, choose smaller plates.
- Listen to Hunger Cues: Recognise your signs of hunger and fullness to prevent overindulging.

11. Involve Caregivers or Family:

- Cook Together: Include family members or carers in meal preparation if at all possible to create a fun and pleasurable shared experience.
- Share Preferences: To guarantee support from others helping with meals, be clear about dietary needs and preferences.

12. Regular Monitoring and Adaptation:

- Monitor Blood Sugar Levels: Check blood sugar readings frequently to learn how dietary decisions affect the management of diabetes.
- Adapt as Needed: Make dietary adjustments based on blood sugar readings and seek advice from medical authorities.

Giving older citizens useful advice on how to include nutrient-dense foods in their regular meals helps them control their diabetes and maintain general health. Encouraging seniors to choose food with awareness, moderation, and diversity allows them to have a varied and nutrient-dense diet that suits their individual needs. For best outcomes, it is advised to get individualized guidance from certified dietitians or medical professionals.

ROLE OF NUTRITION IN MANAGING DIABETES COMPLICATIONS

Nutrition is essential for controlling the problems of diabetes since it has a direct impact on cardiovascular health, blood sugar regulation, and general well-being. A nutrient-rich, well-balanced diet customized to each person's needs can help avoid and treat diabetes-related problems. This is a thorough examination of the role that nutrition plays in managing various issues associated with diabetes:

1. Cardiovascular Complications:

Managing Blood Pressure:

- Reducing Sodium Intake: Reducing sodium intake aids in blood pressure control. Select whole, fresh foods over processed ones.
- Increasing Potassium: Foods high in potassium, such as fruits and vegetables, help to better regulate blood pressure.

Promoting Heart Health:

- Incorporating Omega-3 Fatty Acids: Walnuts, flaxseeds, and fatty fish all improve lipid profiles and lower inflammation, which is beneficial for heart health.
- Emphasizing Healthy Fats: In order to control cholesterol levels, choose monounsaturated and polyunsaturated fats instead of saturated and trans fats.

2. Neuropathy:

Managing Blood Sugar Levels:

- Stabilizing Blood Glucose: A steady diet of carbohydrates spaced out throughout the day helps avoid blood sugar spikes, which can aggravate nerve damage.
- Preventing Severe Highs and Lows: By maintaining blood sugar levels within a specific range, neuropathic problems are less likely to occur.

Antioxidants and Anti-Inflammatory Foods:

- Incorporating Antioxidants: Antioxidant-rich foods including almonds, berries, and dark leafy greens may help lessen oxidative stress, which is linked to neuropathy.
- Anti-Inflammatory Diet: Choosing a diet that lowers inflammation could help with neuropathy symptoms.

3. Nephropathy (Kidney Disease):

Sodium and Fluid Balance:

- Sodium Restriction: Reducing sodium consumption eases the burden on the kidneys by assisting in blood pressure management and fluid balance.
- Adequate Hydration: Renal function is supported by maintaining an appropriate fluid intake.

Protein Management:

Moderating Protein Intake: Reducing protein consumption can help the kidneys work less hard. Select sources of high-quality protein.

4. Retinopathy:

Blood Sugar Control:

- Stable Blood Glucose Levels: The blood vessels in the eyes can be protected from injury by maintaining constant blood sugar levels.
- Consistent Monitoring: Frequent blood sugar testing enables dietary adjustments for the best possible control.

Antioxidant-Rich Foods:

- Protecting Eye Health: Antioxidant-rich foods like berries, carrots, and leafy greens support eye health and may even help prevent retinopathy.

5. Wound Healing:

Protein Intake:

- Adequate Protein: Protein is necessary for wound healing and tissue repair. Make sure you consume enough protein from foods like dairy, lentils, and lean meats.
- Vitamin C-Rich Foods: Vitamin C aids in the synthesis of collagen and the healing of wounds. Add bell peppers, berries, and citrus fruits to your diet.

Maintaining Blood Sugar Control:

- Stable Blood Glucose Levels: Consistent blood sugar control promotes efficient wound healing and reduces the risk of infections.

6. Weight Management:

Balanced Nutrition:

- Portion Control: Controlling portion sizes promotes weight management by assisting with calorie intake control.
- Nutrient-Rich Choices: Selecting foods high in nutrients guarantees the body gets the vital vitamins and minerals it needs.

Physical Activity:

- Caloric Expenditure: Frequent exercise enhances insulin sensitivity and aids in weight management.
- Muscle Maintenance: Maintaining muscle mass with resistance training promotes good metabolic health overall.

7. Gastrointestinal Complications:

Fiber-Rich Diet:

- Digestive Health: Consuming a diet high in fruits, vegetables, and whole grains—which are high in fiber—supports healthy digestion and keeps constipation at bay.
- Blood Sugar Control: Fibre reduces the rate at which glucose is absorbed, which helps regulate blood sugar.

Probiotics:

- Maintaining Gut Health: Probiotics can help with digestive problems and support a healthy gut microbiome. They can be found in yogurt, kefir, and fermented foods.

8. Mental Health:

Nutrient-Rich Foods for Brain Health:

- Omega-3 Fatty Acids: Walnuts, flaxseeds, and fatty fish all promote mental health and cognitive performance.
- Antioxidant-Rich Foods: Dark leafy greens and berries are good sources of antioxidants that may shield the brain from oxidative stress.

Blood Sugar Stability:

- Balanced Meals: Better mental and emotional stability is correlated with stable blood sugar levels.
- Hydration: It's important to stay properly hydrated because dehydration can impair mood and cognitive abilities.

In summary, a nutrient-rich, well-balanced diet is essential for both managing and averting problems related to diabetes. When certain nutrients are included together with an emphasis on blood sugar regulation and general health, people are empowered to take charge of their diabetes care. To ensure that dietary choices are in line with specific health needs and goals, seeking personalized assistance from healthcare professionals or registered dietitians is recommended.

PHYSICAL WELL-BEING

Having a healthy body is important for general health, especially for older adults. Keeping one's body in good condition as one ages is crucial for independence, happiness, and the avoidance of chronic illnesses. This section examines a number of topics related to seniors' physical health, such as the value of consistent exercise, customising physical activity to meet needs, and managing long-term medical issues.

Benefits of Exercise for Diabetes

Frequent exercise has numerous advantages for people with diabetes that affect both mental and physical health. we shall examine the benefits of exercise, including:

- Enhanced Cardiovascular Health: improving circulation and heart health.
- Maintained Mobility and Flexibility: Avoiding stiffness and maintaining joint function.
- Strengthened Muscles and Bones: Lowering the chance of fractures and falls.
- Cognitive Benefits: Promoting mental clarity and lowering the likelihood of cognitive deterioration.
- Mood Improvement: Improving mental health and lowering depressive and anxious feelings.

Types of Suitable Exercises for Diabetes

Cardiovascular Exercises: Walking, swimming, and cycling are examples of mild aerobic exercises.

Strength Training: Embrace resistance training to preserve muscular mass.

Flexibility and Balance Exercises: Exercises for balance and stretching to avoid falls.

Low-Impact Options: Gentle exercises for the joints, such tai chi or yoga.

Overcoming Barriers to Exercise

There can be particular difficulties you encounter when exercising. This section will address doable methods for getting beyond obstacles, such as:

- Adapting Exercises: Adjusting activities based on each person's capabilities and health.
- Incorporating Daily Activity: Encouraging light physical activity all day long.
- Social Engagement: Taking part in exercises or activities with others in the group for company and incentive.
- Consulting Healthcare Professionals: Asking medical professionals for advice on individualised fitness regimens.

Tailoring Exercise Routines for Seniors
Individualized Exercise Plans

- The significance of developing customised exercise regimens based on goals, preferences, and health status is emphasised in this paragraph. Topics cover:
- Health Assessment: Carrying out a thorough evaluation to ascertain fitness levels and pinpoint possible hazards.
- Setting Realistic Goals: Setting attainable short- and long-term objectives will help to increase motivation.
- Modifying Routines: Workout regimens should be modified as abilities or health problems evolve.

- Incorporating Variety: Incorporating a range of workouts to maintain a dynamic and captivating regimen.

Incorporating Exercise into Daily Life

- Promoting people to incorporate physical activity into their everyday routines is essential. The strategies covered in this section include:
- Functional Exercises: Concentrating on motions that resemble everyday tasks for useful advantages.
- Creating a Routine: Establishing a regular workout schedule in order to form habits.
- Utilizing Everyday Items: Using household things for resistance training.
- Prioritizing Safety: Ensuring that workout spaces are secure and appropriate for each individual.

MANAGING CHRONIC CONDITIONS THROUGH PHYSICAL ACTIVITY

Diabetes Management through Exercise

- Blood Sugar Regulation: How exercise contributes to blood glucose stabilisation.
- Consulting Healthcare Providers: The significance of consulting a physician for specific exercise recommendations.
- Preventing Complications: Engaging in physical activity can help avert issues associated with diabetes.

Arthritis and Joint Health

People frequently struggle with arthritis, which limits their movement:

- Low-Impact Exercises: Gentle exercises to keep joints flexible without making discomfort worse.
- Aquatic Exercise: The advantages of water-based exercises for healthy joints.
- Pain Management Strategies: Including workouts that reduce joint pain instead of making it worse.

Cardiovascular Exercise for Heart Health

Exercise is essential for people with cardiovascular diseases. Vital details consist of:

Moderate Intensity Exercises: taking part in low-stress activities that support cardiovascular health.

Monitoring Intensity: Determining the intensity of an exercise routine by heart rate monitoring or perceived effort.

Gradual Progression: The significance of escalating exercise intensity gradually after a cautious start.

In summary, encouraging regular exercise, customising routines to meet individual needs, and managing chronic health issues through physical activity are all important aspects of fostering physical well-being in seniors. Seniors' general health is improved by a comprehensive approach to physical well-being, which helps them to keep their independence and enjoy happy lives.

INCORPORATING FIBER AND WHOLE GRAINS INTO YOUR DIET

Whole grains and fibre are vital parts of a balanced diet and provide several health advantages, particularly for those with diabetes. Including these ingredients in your meals can help maintain healthy digestion, control blood sugar, and improve general wellbeing. Here's how to incorporate whole grains and fibre into your diet on a regular basis:

1. Start Your Day with Whole Grains:

- Whole Grain Cereals: Select cereals where the main constituent is whole grains. Seek products with the fewest amount of added sugar.
- Oatmeal: For maximum taste and nutrition, use steel-cut or rolled oats and top with your preferred fruits or nuts.

2. Choose Whole Grain Bread:

- Whole Wheat Bread: For sandwiches and toast, use whole wheat or whole grain bread instead.
- Look for Labels: Make sure the item identified as "whole wheat" or "whole grain" comes first.

3. Embrace Quinoa:

- Quinoa: For a nutrient-dense, whole grain substitute, try quinoa instead of rice or pasta.
- Versatile: Quinoa may be a great addition to salads, side dishes, and meals high in protein.

4. Snack on Whole Grain Crackers:

- Whole Grain Crackers: For a filling snack, pair whole grain crackers with cheese, hummus, or your preferred nut butter.
- Check Ingredients: Make sure the crackers are made of nutritious grains and don't have any bad fats or a lot of added sugar.

5. Add Barley to Soups and Stews:

- Barley: Barley is a hearty, high-fiber component to soups and stews.
- Cooking Tip: For extra flavour, cook barley in vegetable or chicken broth.

6. Experiment with Bulgur:

- Bulgur: Use bulgur as a filling for vegetables or to make salads and pilafs. This whole grain has a nutty flavour and cooks quickly.
- High in Fiber: Bulgur gives your food texture and is a wonderful source of fibre.

7. Snack on Popcorn:

- Air-Popped Popcorn: Treat yourself to whole grain popcorn that has been air-popped. Herbs or nutritional yeast can be added for flavour instead of butter.
- Portion Control: To maintain the snack's healthfulness, watch the portion quantities.

8. Include Whole Grains in Pasta Dishes:

- Whole Grain Pasta: Choose whole grain or whole wheat pasta for your favorite pasta dishes.
- Pair with Veggies: To increase the fibre and nutrients in your pasta, add a lot of vegetables.

9. Mix Whole Grains in Salads:

- Quinoa or Farro Salads: Make salads by starting with quinoa or farro and then adding vibrant veggies, lean meats, and a mild vinaigrette.
- Prep in Advance: Make a large batch of whole grain salads for wholesome, easy-to-make dinners all week long.

10. Choose Brown Rice:

- Brown Rice: If you want to use entire grains, go for brown rice rather than white rice.
- Variety: Try experimenting with other types of brown rice, including jasmine or basmati.

11. Blend Whole Grains into Smoothies:

- Oats or Barley Flakes: To up the fibre content of your morning smoothie, stir in a scoop of oats or barley flakes.
- Blend with Fruits: Blend with yoghurt, fruits, and your preferred liquid to make a wholesome and satisfying beverage.

12. Snack on Whole Grain Granola:

- Whole Grain Granola: Select whole grain, almond, and seed granola for a satisfyingly crispy snack.
- Pair with Yogurt: Savour it as a fruit topping or with yoghurt.

13. Explore Whole Grain Wraps:

- Whole Grain Wraps or Tortillas: For a healthier option, use whole grain wraps instead of normal wraps.
- Filled with Veggies: Stuff your wraps with of vibrant veggies and lean meats.

14. Bake with Whole Grain Flour:

- Whole Wheat Flour: Try adding more fibre to your baking recipes by experimenting with whole wheat flour.
- Combine Flours: Make a gradual switch to whole wheat flour in your recipes from refined flour.

15. Read Food Labels:

Check for Whole Grains: When you go grocery shopping, look for products labelled "whole grains." Search for phrases such as "brown rice," "whole wheat," or "whole oats."

It's not difficult to include whole grains and fibre in your everyday meals. Make these adjustments gradually, try out various solutions, and determine which suits your tastes the best. The variety of whole grains and foods high in fibre provides a wealth of mouthwatering options for preparing meals that are both balanced and nourishing.

BENEFITS OF FIBER FOR DIABETES

A diet that is diabetes-friendly must include fibre since it provides a number of health advantages that promote blood sugar regulation and general wellbeing. The following are the main advantages of adding fibre to the diet for people with diabetes:

1. Blood Sugar Regulation:

Stabilizing Blood Glucose Levels: Consumed in foods such as fruits, beans, and oats, soluble fibre slows down the absorption of glucose by forming a gel-like substance that helps to keep blood sugar levels steady.

2. Improved Insulin Sensitivity:

Enhancing Insulin Function: Foods high in fibre may increase sensitivity to insulin, enhancing the uptake of glucose into cells and enabling cells to react to insulin more efficiently.

3. Weight Management:

Promoting Satiety: Because high-fiber foods are frequently more filling, they can aid in weight management, which is important for people with diabetes and help regulate hunger.

4. Cardiovascular Health:

Lowering Cholesterol Levels: By reducing LDL (low-density lipoprotein) cholesterol, soluble fibre supports heart health and lowers the risk of diabetes-related cardiovascular problems.

5. Digestive Health:

Preventing Constipation: Because insoluble fibre gives the stool more volume, it encourages regular bowel movements and helps people avoid constipation, which is a major problem for many diabetics.

6. Blood Pressure Control:

Supporting Healthy Blood Pressure: Some fibres, especially those present in fruits, vegetables, and whole grains, have the potential to reduce blood pressure.

7. Slow Absorption of Carbohydrates:

Managing Post-Meal Spikes: Fibre helps avoid sharp rises in blood sugar levels after meals by slowing down the breakdown and absorption of carbohydrates.

8. Blood Lipid Management:

Triglyceride Reduction: Triglyceride levels may be lowered with the aid of fibre, improving lipid profiles and lowering the risk of cardiovascular problems.

9. Promoting Gut Health:

Feeding Beneficial Gut Bacteria: Certain fibres support a healthy gut microbiome and nourish good gut bacteria since they are prebiotics.

10. Long-term Blood Sugar Control: Improvement in HbA1c: Regular consumption of foods high in fibre has been linked to improvements in HbA1c readings, which are a measure of long-term blood sugar control.

FIBER-RICH RECIPES FOR DIABETICS:

Including fibre in meals can be tasty and advantageous for those with diabetes. The following recipes, which are high in fibre and appropriate for people with diabetes, include:

1. Overnight Oats with Berries:

Ingredients:

- Rolled oats
- Greek yogurt
- Berries (blueberries, strawberries)
- Chia seeds

Instructions:

- Mix oats, yogurt, berries, and chia seeds in a jar.
- Refrigerate overnight and enjoy a fiber-packed breakfast.

2. Quinoa Salad with Vegetables:

Ingredients:

- Cooked quinoa
- Mixed vegetables (bell peppers, cucumbers, cherry tomatoes)
- Olive oil and lemon dressing
- Feta cheese (optional)

Instructions:

- Combine cooked quinoa with chopped vegetables.
- Drizzle with olive oil and lemon dressing, toss, and top with feta if desired.

3. Lentil Soup:

Ingredients:

- Lentils
- Vegetables (carrots, celery, onions)
- Low-sodium vegetable broth
- Garlic and spices

Instructions:

- Sauté vegetables, add lentils, broth, and spices.
- Simmer until lentils are tender for a hearty, fiber-rich soup.

4. Whole Grain Wraps with Grilled Chicken:

Ingredients:

- Whole grain wraps
- Grilled chicken strips

- Mixed greens
- Hummus or Greek yogurt dressing

Instructions:

Top whole grain wrappers with Greek yoghurt dressing or hummus, grilled chicken, and mixed greens.

5. Roasted Vegetable Medley:

Ingredients:

- Assorted vegetables (zucchini, bell peppers, cherry tomatoes)
- Olive oil and herbs

Instructions:

- Toss vegetables in olive oil and herbs, roast until tender.
- Serve as a fiber-rich side dish or over quinoa.

6. Berry Smoothie with Flaxseeds:

Ingredients:

- Mixed berries (strawberries, raspberries, blueberries)
- Greek yogurt
- Almond milk
- Ground flaxseeds

Instructions:

- Blend berries, yogurt, almond milk, and flaxseeds for a nutritious and fiber-rich smoothie.

7. Stir-fried Broccoli and Tofu:

Ingredients:

- Broccoli florets
- Tofu cubes
- Soy sauce
- Garlic and ginger

Instructions:

Tofu and broccoli can be stir-fried with garlic, ginger, and a small amount of soy sauce to provide a quick and high-fiber lunch.

Don't forget to speak with a medical expert or a qualified dietitian to make sure these recipes suit your specific dietary requirements and your diabetes control objectives.

LEAN PROTEINS AND HEALTHY FATS

Including lean proteins and healthy fats in diabetes control is crucial for preserving blood sugar levels, fostering heart health, and guaranteeing general wellbeing. In addition to discussing the significance of various macronutrients, this section provides helpful advice on how to include them in a balanced diet.

Importance of Lean Proteins:

1. Blood Sugar Regulation:

- Lean proteins help regulate blood sugar levels by releasing energy steadily and having little effect on blood sugar levels.
- Lean protein consumption at meals reduces the risk of abrupt blood glucose rises and falls.

2. Satiety and Weight Management:

- Proteins contribute to a feeling of fullness and satisfaction, supporting weight management by reducing overall food intake.
- Sustained satiety helps prevent overeating and promotes a balanced and controlled approach to meals.

3. Muscle Maintenance and Repair:

Sufficient consumption of protein is essential for preserving muscle mass, facilitating tissue regeneration, and averting muscular atrophy, particularly in the case of diabetes.

Examples of Lean Proteins:

1. Poultry:

- Turkey or chicken breasts without skin.
- Baked or grilled foods reduce additional fats.

2. Fish:

- Omega-3-rich fatty fish, such as mackerel, trout, and salmon.
- Lean alternatives, like fish or tilapia.

3. Plant-Based Proteins:

- legumes such as black beans, chickpeas, and lentils.
- Edamame, tofu, and tempeh are flexible plant-based protein sources.

4. Lean Cuts of Meat:

- Steaks that are lean, like tenderloin or sirloin.
- Trimmed pork loin chops or tenderloin to remove any visible fat.

5. Dairy and Eggs:

- Dairy products with reduced or no fat, such as cottage cheese or Greek yoghurt.
- Eggs are a high-nutrient protein source.

Importance of Healthy Fats:

1. Heart Health:

- Good fats, especially those that are mono- and polyunsaturated, lower LDL cholesterol and triglyceride levels, which promote cardiovascular health.
- Their contribution results in a decreased risk of heart disease, which is a significant concern among people with diabetes.

2. Blood Sugar Regulation:

- Stable blood sugar levels are supported by healthy fats because they slow down the absorption of carbs.
- Meals high in fat can help reduce the likelihood of sharp increases in blood sugar levels after eating.

3. Nutrient Absorption:

- Fats help guarantee that the body gets the necessary nutrients by assisting in the absorption of fat-soluble vitamins (A, D, E, and K).

Examples of Healthy Fats:

1. Avocado:

Avocados are high in monounsaturated fats and add a creamy texture and variety of nutrients to dishes.

2. Olive Oil:

A mainstay of the Mediterranean diet, extra virgin olive oil provides antioxidants and monounsaturated fats.

3. Nuts and Seeds:

A combination of fibre, necessary minerals, and good fats can be found in almonds, walnuts, chia seeds, and flaxseeds.

4. Fatty Fish:

High-quality protein and omega-3 fatty acids can be found in abundance in salmon, mackerel, and sardines.

5 Nut Butters:

You may put cashew, almond, or natural peanut butter on whole grain toast or blend it into smoothies.

Practical Tips for Incorporating Lean Proteins and Healthy Fats:

1. Balanced Meals:

Make sure your meals are well-balanced with plenty of colourful veggies, complete grains, lean meats, and healthy fats.

2. Portion Control:

Even if fats are healthful, portion control is a good way to keep calories in check and avoid consuming too much of them.

3. Cooking Methods:

To maintain the nutritional value of proteins and lipids, opt for healthy cooking techniques like grilling, baking, steaming, or sautéing with little to no oil.

4. Snack Smart:

To stay full in between meals, choose nutrient-dense snacks like Greek yoghurt or a handful of nuts.

5. Diverse Protein Sources:

To guarantee a diversity of nutrients and avoid nutritional boredom, switch up your protein sources.

6 Read Labels:

When buying packaged foods, check the labels to find sources of lean proteins and healthy fats. You should also be aware of any added sugars or harmful ingredients.

A diabetes-friendly diet that includes lean proteins and healthy fats is essential for controlling blood sugar levels and enhancing general health. For those with diabetes, these macronutrients can help with satiety, weight control, and cardiovascular health when they are carefully selected and taken in the right amounts. Personalised advice based on dietary preferences and unique health requirements can be obtained by speaking with a licenced dietitian or other healthcare expert.

PROTEIN REQUIREMENTS FOR DIABETES AFTER 60

Maintaining a sufficient protein intake as people age is essential for immune system support, muscular mass preservation, and general health. Knowing the amount of protein required is crucial for anyone treating diabetes after the age of 60. This section examines the protein requirements of elderly individuals with diabetes and provides recommendations for including foods high in protein in their diet.

Protein Requirements:

1. Preserving Muscle Mass:

There is a natural decrease in muscle mass that comes with ageing. Sufficient consumption of protein helps prevent muscular atrophy and enhances strength and range of motion.

2. Immune Function:

Proteins are essential for sustaining a strong immune system, which helps the body fend against diseases and infections.

3. Blood Sugar Control:

Because protein slows down the absorption of carbohydrates, it helps to stabilise blood sugar levels throughout meals.

Sources of Healthy Fats

Healthy fats should be the main focus of a diabetic's diet in order to promote heart health and general wellbeing. This section focuses on sources of good fats that are appropriate for those over 60 who are controlling their diabetes.

1. Avocado:

Avocados are a great source of critical minerals and heart-healthy monounsaturated fats.

2. Olive Oil:

A mainstay of the Mediterranean diet, extra virgin olive oil provides antioxidants and monounsaturated fats.

3. Nuts and Seeds:

A combination of fibre, necessary minerals, and good fats can be found in almonds, walnuts, chia seeds, and flaxseeds.

4. Fatty Fish:

Sardines, mackerel, and salmon are great providers of high-quality protein and omega-3 fatty acids.

5. Nut Butters:

You may put cashew, almond, or natural peanut butter on whole grain toast or blend it into smoothies.

Cooking Techniques for Heart-Healthy Meals

Seniors with diabetes must learn heart-healthy cooking habits in order to maintain their cardiovascular health. This section looks at cooking techniques that promote general health and maintain the nutritional value of ingredients.

1. Grilling:

Flavour is imparted by grilling without using a lot of extra fat. For a well-rounded dinner, choose lean proteins like fish or chicken and add veggies.

2. Baking:

Baking uses little additional fat and is a heart-healthy choice. For a wholesome dinner, prepare items like baked fish, poultry, or veggies.

3. Steaming:

Foods' inherent flavours and nutrients can be preserved with steaming, negating the need for additional lipids. For a nutritious and light supper, try steaming whole grains, fish, or vegetables.

4. Sautéing with Healthy Oils:

When sautéing, use heart-healthy oils like avocado or olive oil. To make this dish tasty, add lean proteins and a variety of vegetables.

5. Roasting:

Tofu, lean meats, and veggies all taste better when roasted while retaining their nutritious value. Incorporate spices and herbs for flavour.

6. Slow Cooking:

Flavours can combine through slow cooking without using a lot of additional fat. Make lean protein, vegetable, and whole grain stews or soups.

7. Portion Control:

To control calorie consumption, use portion control. To assist in providing portions that are acceptable, use smaller bowls and plates.

After the age of 60, seniors with diabetes must incorporate heart-friendly cooking techniques, adequate protein, and healthy fats. These dietary factors support cardiovascular health, blood sugar regulation, and general health. Since every person's needs are different, speaking with medical specialists or registered dietitians is advised for individualised advice and nutrition regimens catered to certain health issues and objectives.

MANAGING CARBOHYDRATES FOR DIABETES AFTER 60

A crucial component of treating diabetes, particularly in people over 60, is controlling carbs. This section explores the significance of managing carbs, provides helpful hints for selecting the appropriate kinds and quantities of carbohydrates, and offers information on how seniors with diabetes can keep their blood sugar under control.

Importance of Carbohydrate Management:

1. Blood Sugar Control:

In order to stabilise blood sugar levels, avoid hyperglycemia, and reduce the risk of complications from diabetes, proper management of carbohydrates is essential.

2. Energy Source:

The body uses carbs as its main energy source. A consistent and regulated release of glucose to support everyday activities is ensured by effective management.

3. Individualized Approach:

Individuals with diabetes should control their carbohydrate intake individually based on their activity level, medications, and general health.

Practical Tips for Choosing Carbohydrates:

1. Emphasize Whole Grains:

For more fibre and nutrients, choose whole grains like quinoa, brown rice, and whole wheat bread instead than processed grains.

2. Include High-Fiber Foods:

To slow down the absorption of glucose and support digestive health, include foods high in fibre, such as fruits, vegetables, legumes, and whole grains.

3. Watch Portion Sizes:

Pay attention to portion proportions to prevent consuming too many carbohydrates. Make use of measurement devices and become acquainted with the suggested portion sizes.

4. Prioritize Complex Carbohydrates:

Pay attention to complex carbs like sweet potatoes, beans, and lentils that provide you energy for a long time.

5. Limit Added Sugars:

Reduce the amount of added-sugar foods and beverages you consume. When satiating a sweet tooth, go for fruits' inherent sweetness.

Timing and Distribution of Carbohydrates:

1. Spread Carbohydrates Throughout the Day:

To prevent blood sugar spikes and crashes, divide your carbohydrate intake equally between meals and snacks.

2. Consider Glycemic Index:

Understand the glycemic index (GI) of the foods you eat. Selecting low-GI foods can aid in better blood sugar control.

3. Monitor Blood Sugar Levels:

Keep an eye on your blood sugar levels to see how various carbs affect different reactions in people.

Individualized Meal Planning:

1. Consult with a Dietitian:

Create a customised meal plan with the help of a trained dietician based on your preferences, lifestyle, and health requirements.

2. Consider Medication Timing:

To achieve optimal blood sugar control, synchronise your consumption of carbohydrates with your prescription schedule. Seek advice from medical professionals.

3. Adjust Based on Activity Levels:

Adapt your carbohydrate intake to your degree of physical activity. To sustain energy levels after or before exercise, think about include a snack.

Smart Snacking:

1. Choose Nutrient-Dense Snacks:

Choose nutrient-dense snacks such as raw veggies with hummus, Greek yoghurt, or a tiny handful of nuts.

2. Combine Carbohydrates with Protein:

For well-balanced snacks that help control blood sugar levels and offer prolonged energy, pair carbohydrates with protein.

3. Read Food Labels:

To find out the amount of fibre, added sugars, and total carbohydrates in a food, read the labels. Making educated decisions during grocery shopping is aided by this.

Effective carbohydrate management is essential to elder diabetic care. People over 60 can optimise blood sugar control, boost energy levels, and promote general well-being by practising mindful carbohydrate selection, portion restriction, and personalised meal planning. Maintaining effective diabetes treatment requires regular discussion with healthcare providers, particularly dietitians, to make sure dietary decisions support personal health objectives.

UNDERSTANDING GLYCEMIC INDEX

The GI, or glycemic index, gauges how rapidly a diet high in carbohydrates boosts blood sugar levels. Foods can have GI values of low, medium, or high.

1. Impact on Blood Sugar:

Low-GI foods result in a slower, more steady rise in blood sugar levels, whereas high-GI foods induce a sudden spike. Having a thorough understanding of the GI can empower people to regulate their blood sugar in an informed manner.

2. Incorporating Low-GI Foods:

Choose low-GI foods such as whole grains, legumes, and non-starchy vegetables to promote stable blood sugar levels over time.

Smart Carbohydrate Choices:

1. Whole Grains:

If you want more nutrients and longer-lasting energy, choose whole grains like quinoa, brown rice, and whole wheat bread over processed grains.

2. Colorful Vegetables:

Incorporate a range of vibrant, non-starchy vegetables into your meals. They have less of an effect on blood sugar and are high in fibre, vitamins, and minerals.

3. Legumes and Pulses:

As great providers of both fibre and protein, beans, lentils, and chickpeas are wise options for maintaining stable blood sugar levels.

4. Berries:

Strawberries and blueberries are two berries that are rich in antioxidants and low in sugar. They naturally sweeten food without significantly raising blood sugar levels.

5. Nuts and Seeds:

Add almonds, chia seeds, and flaxseeds to your diet to get a mix of fibre, protein, and healthy fats.

Balancing Carbohydrates for Stable Blood Sugar:

1. Portion Control:

To control your intake of carbohydrates, practise portion management. Consider portion proportions to prevent overindulging.

2. Combine with Protein:

To help stabilise blood sugar levels and slow down the absorption of glucose, combine carbs with lean protein.

3. Include Healthy Fats:

By slowing down the absorption of carbs, adding healthy fats like avocado or olive oil to meals helps maintain blood sugar stability.

4. Regular Meal Timing:

Try to eat at regular times to keep your energy levels stable and avoid significant blood sugar swings.

5. Snack Wisely:

To maintain stable blood sugar levels in between meals, choose balanced snacks that include protein, healthy fats, and carbohydrates.

6. Hydration:

Drink plenty of water because dehydration might lower blood sugar. Drink water or herbal teas instead of sugar-filled drinks.

Individualized Approach:

1. Consult with Healthcare Professionals:

Collaborate closely with medical specialists, such as diabetes educators and dietitians, to create a customised carbohydrate management strategy based on your unique health objectives.

2. Regular Monitoring:

Keep an eye on your blood sugar levels and modify your carbohydrate consumption in accordance with your doctor's advice and personal responses.

Making wise decisions, striking the correct balance, and comprehending the glycemic index are all necessary for managing carbohydrates effectively. Seniors with diabetes can maintain stable blood sugar levels and promote overall well-being by consuming low-GI foods, selecting nutrient-dense options, and combining carbohydrates with protein and healthy fats. Tailored advice from medical specialists guarantees that food plans meet specific health requirements and help with effective diabetes control.

HYDRATION AND DIABETES

An essential component of managing diabetes is staying properly hydrated, which also supports ideal blood sugar control and general health. This section examines the importance of staying hydrated for people with diabetes, offers recommendations for consuming the right amount of fluids, and emphasises the effects of staying hydrated on a number of different elements of wellbeing.

Importance of Hydration:

1. Blood Sugar Regulation:

Sufficient hydration promotes renal function, which is essential for excreting excess glucose through urine and helps control blood sugar levels.

2. Prevention of Dehydration:

Elevations in blood sugar levels may result from dehydration. Keeping fluid levels adequate helps avoid dehydration and the possible effects it may have on blood sugar.

3. Digestive Health:

Drinking enough water promotes healthy digestion and nutrition absorption, which benefits overall digestive health, which is especially important for those with diabetes.

4. Temperature Regulation:

In order to assist the body adjust to its surroundings and avoid heat-related problems, hydration is essential for temperature control.

5. Cardiovascular Health:

Because well-hydrated blood is easier for the heart to pump, cardiovascular health is promoted. This is important to take into account for diabetics, as they may be more susceptible to heart-related problems.

Guidelines for Hydration:

1. Daily Water Intake:

Because well-hydrated blood is easier for the heart to pump, cardiovascular health is promoted. This is important to take into account for diabetics, as they may be more susceptible to heart-related problems.

2. Spread Intake Throughout the Day:

Because well-hydrated blood is easier for the heart to pump, cardiovascular health is promoted. This is important to take into account for diabetics, as they may be more susceptible to heart-related problems.

3 Consider Other Fluid Sources:

Use additional sources of hydration, like herbal teas, infused water, and broths, to increase the amount of fluids consumed overall and to provide taste and diversity.

4. Monitor Thirst Levels:

Observe signs of thirst. The body naturally senses thirst as a sign that it needs to be hydrated. In order to preserve ideal fluid equilibrium, act quickly.

Impact of Hydration on Medication:

1. Influence on Medication Absorption:

Maintaining adequate water facilitates the assimilation of prescribed diabetes drugs, guaranteeing their efficient absorption for the best possible blood sugar regulation.

2. Interaction with Diuretics:

Dehydration may result from the increased urine production caused by some diabetes treatments, especially diuretics. To counteract the effects of these medications, it is imperative to stay hydrated.

Hydration and Physical Activity:

1. Pre-Exercise Hydration:

Be sure to hydrate well before engaging in any physical activity. Consuming enough fluids increases endurance and prevents dehydration during exercise.

2. During Exercise:

Be sure to hydrate well before engaging in any physical activity. Consuming enough fluids increases endurance and prevents dehydration during exercise.

Monitoring Hydration Status:

1. Urine Color:

Use urine colour as a straightforward gauge of your level of hydration. While dark yellow or amber urine may indicate dehydration, pale yellow pee often indicates appropriate hydration.

2. Individual Factors:

Take into account personal characteristics like age, health, and environment when determining hydration requirements. Diabetes sufferers may need to modify their hydration regimens in light of particular medical concerns.

Challenges and Solutions:

1. Increased Thirst from Medications:

Certain diabetes drugs may make you feel more thirsty. Work with medical professionals in these situations to balance the effects of medication with enough fluids.

2. Fluid Restrictions:

When some medical problems limit your ability to consume fluids, work with medical providers to create a hydration strategy that complies with recommendations while keeping you well hydrated.

A key element of managing diabetes is staying hydrated, which affects blood sugar regulation as well as general health and wellbeing. People with diabetes can improve their health outcomes and help ensure successful diabetes care by taking a proactive hydration regimen. Since everyone's demands for hydration differ, speaking with medical professionals—registered dietitians among them—ensures that hydration regimens are tailored to the needs of the individual and in line with particular health objectives.

BEST BEVERAGE CHOICES FOR SENIOR DIABETICS

Selecting the appropriate drinks is crucial for elderly people with diabetes since it has an immediate effect on blood sugar levels and general health. The best beverage options for elderly people with diabetes are discussed in this area, with a focus on selections that help with blood sugar regulation and hydration.

1. Water:

Benefits:

- Pure and calorie-free.
- Supports optimal hydration.
- Essential for various bodily functions.

Tips:

- Keep a reusable water bottle with you to promote consistent water consumption.
- Slices of cucumber or citrus fruit can be added to water to give it flavour without adding any more sugar.

2. Herbal Teas:

Benefits:

- Non-caffeinated.
- Various flavors available.
- May have additional health benefits, depending on the herbs used.

Tips:

- To avoid extra sugars, choose herbal teas that aren't sweetened.
- Try a variety of herbal mixtures by experimenting.

3. Green Tea:

Benefits:

- Contains antioxidants.
- Potential benefits for heart health.
- Moderate caffeine content.

Tips:

- If you have a caffeine sensitivity, go for decaffeinated green tea.
- Savour it without any added flavouring or with a squeeze of lemon.

4. Sparkling Water:

Benefits:

- Calorie-free.
- Provides a fizzy, refreshing option.

- Available in various flavors.

Tips:

- Pick sparkling water that isn't sweetened or that is just plain.
- For a touch of sweetness, add a dash of organic fruit juice.

5. Vegetable Juice:

Benefits:

- Rich in vitamins and minerals.
- Lower in sugar compared to fruit juices.
- Can be a convenient way to incorporate vegetables.

Tips:

- Choose low-sodium varieties.
- Consider diluting with water to reduce overall sugar content.

6. Low-Fat Milk:

Benefits:

- Good source of calcium and vitamin D.
- Provides protein.
- Moderately low in carbohydrates.

Tips:

- Opt for low-fat or skim milk to reduce saturated fat intake.
- Watch portion sizes to manage calorie and carbohydrate intake.

7. Coconut Water:

Benefits:

- Naturally hydrating.
- Contains electrolytes.
- Low in calories and fat.

Tips:

- Choose plain coconut water without added sugars.
- Consume in moderation due to natural sugars.

8. Coffee:

Benefits:

- Rich in antioxidants.
- May have potential health benefits.
- Low in calories.

Tips:

- Limit added sugars and high-fat creamers.

- Be mindful of caffeine intake, especially in the afternoon.

9. Infused Water:

Benefits:

Adds natural flavor without added sugars.

- Encourages increased water intake.
- Can include various fruits, herbs, and even vegetables.

Tips:

- Experiment with different combinations like cucumber-mint or berry-citrus.

10. Unsweetened Almond Milk:

Benefits:

- Low in carbohydrates.
- Suitable for those with lactose intolerance.
- May contain added vitamins and minerals.

Tips:

- Choose unsweetened varieties to avoid added sugars.
- Check for fortified options for added nutritional benefits.

HYDRATION TIPS FOR DIABETICS

Staying well hydrated is especially important for elderly people with diabetes. This section offers helpful advice on how to stay properly hydrated while taking into account the special requirements and difficulties faced by elderly people with diabetes.

1. Regular Monitoring:

- To learn how hydration levels may affect glucose regulation, regularly check blood sugar levels.

2. Spread Intake Throughout the Day:

- Drink liquids frequently during the day to stay as hydrated as possible.

3. Medication Considerations:

- Diabetes drugs should be considered as they may affect hydration and fluid balance. Seek advice from medical professionals.

4. Choose Low-Glycemic Options:

Drinks with a low glycemic index will have less of an effect on blood sugar levels.

5. Limit Sugary Drinks:

Sugar-filled drinks should be avoided as they might cause sharp rises in blood sugar. Select choices free of added sugar.

6. Consider Temperature:

Since seniors may be more vulnerable to heat-related problems, it is important to boost fluid intake during hot weather to prevent dehydration.

7. Address Dental Health:

Select drinks that are kind to your teeth. After ingesting acidic or sugary beverages, rinse your mouth or brush your teeth.

8. Consult with Healthcare Professionals:

Collaborate together with medical professionals, such as dietitians, to develop a customised hydration regimen that meets each person's needs and objectives.

You can promote general health, blood sugar control, and well-being by choosing wisely what to drink and paying attention to senior diabetic hydration guidelines. Maintaining regular contact with medical specialists guarantees that hydration regimens are tailored to specific health needs and help with the effective control of diabetes.

MEAL TIMING AND FREQUENCY FOR DIABETES MANAGEMENT

For those with diabetes, meal timing and frequency are very important in controlling blood sugar levels. The importance of meal timing and frequency is examined in this section, along with tips for developing disciplined eating habits that promote stable glucose control.

Importance of Meal Timing:

1. Blood Sugar Regulation:

Timing meals carefully reduces the risk of severe blood sugar rises and crashes.

2. Insulin Sensitivity:

Meal timing that is optimal increases insulin sensitivity, which improves the body's ability to use insulin to control blood sugar.

3. Energy Distribution:

Eating at regular intervals throughout the day guarantees a steady flow of energy, promoting general wellbeing.

Structured Eating Patterns:

1. Regular Meal Times:

To develop a routine that is in sync with the body's inherent circadian cycle, set regular eating times.

2. Balanced Meals:

At each meal, aim to balance the amounts of healthy fats, proteins, and carbs to help maintain stable blood sugar levels.

3. Snacking Wisely:

Include wholesome snacks in between meals to control energy levels and avoid overindulging in hunger.

Meal Frequency Guidelines:

1. Three Main Meals:

Try to have three well-balanced main meals (lunch, supper, and breakfast) to help you consume fewer calories and get important nutrients.

2. Healthy Snacks:

Between meals, have one or two healthful snacks to help control your blood sugar levels and reduce appetite.

3. Avoid Prolonged Fasting:

To avoid hypoglycemia (low blood sugar) and abnormal glucose patterns, avoid going extended periods without eating.

Meal Timing Strategies:

1. Breakfast:

Eat a healthy meal within an hour of waking up to boost your metabolism and control your blood sugar.

2. Lunch:

Eat a nutritious lunch at noon to maintain your energy levels and avoid overindulging in the afternoon.

3. Dinner:

Choose a lighter meal at least two to three hours before going to bed in order to facilitate digestion and prevent any blood sugar swings during the night.

Considerations for Special Situations:

1. Exercise Timing:

Plan your meals around your workouts, making an effort to eat a healthy meal or snack both before and after.

2. Medication Timing:

Schedule meals to coincide with when you take your prescriptions, particularly if any of them call for food consumption.

3. Social Situations:

When attending social events, make sure your meal plans take your nutritional preferences and goals into account.

Individualized Approach:

1. Consult with Healthcare Professionals:

In close collaboration with healthcare professionals, such as diabetes educators and nutritionists, create a customised meal schedule based on your unique health objectives.

2. Monitor Blood Sugar Responses:

Keep an eye on your blood sugar levels to learn how the time of meals affects each person's glucose reaction.

Hydration with Meals:

1. Importance of Hydration:

During meals, drink plenty of water to facilitate digestion and assist you avoid overindulging.

2. Choose Low-Calorie Beverages:

When drinking with meals, choose water or other low-calorie beverages rather as sweet ones that may affect blood sugar levels.

For diabetics, eating at the right times and in moderation is crucial to controlling blood sugar levels. Optimising glucose management and improving general well-being can be achieved by the adoption of scheduled eating patterns, combining balanced meals and snacks, and taking individual health factors into consideration. Frequent consultation with medical experts guarantees that meal scheduling plans support effective diabetes control and are in line with personal health objectives.

IMPACT OF TIMING ON BLOOD SUGAR

Comprehending the correlation between meal timing and blood sugar levels is imperative for proficient control of diabetes. This section examines how time affects blood sugar levels and offers information on how meal and snack schedules can affect glucose regulation.

Postprandial Blood Sugar:

The term "postprandial blood sugar" describes blood glucose readings obtained following a meal or snack.

1. Peaks and Declines:

Postprandial blood sugar peaks are directly influenced by meal timing. Blood glucose rises in response to carbohydrate consumption; levels peak one to two hours after eating and then progressively decrease.

Breakfast and Morning Blood Sugar:

1. Kickstarting the Day:

Within an hour of waking up, eating a healthy breakfast helps boost metabolism and provide a stable blood sugar baseline for the day.

2. Impact on Insulin Sensitivity:

Eating breakfast has been linked to increased insulin sensitivity, which may result in better blood sugar regulation.

Lunch and Afternoon Blood Sugar:

1. Midday Meal Impact:

A healthy lunch around midday helps maintain energy levels and reduces the risk of noticeable blood sugar swings in the afternoon.

2. Avoiding Overeating:

It's important to eat lunch in order to prevent overindulging during other meals and snacks.

Dinner and Evening Blood Sugar:

1. Lighter Evening Meals:

Choosing a lighter meal at least two to three hours before to going to bed will help prevent blood sugar fluctuations during the night.

2. Impact on Overnight Levels:

When evening meals are planned appropriately, blood sugar stays steady throughout the night and lowers the chance of hyperglycemia in the morning.

Snacking and Blood Sugar:

1. Curbing Hunger:

Healthy between-meal snacks help control blood sugar levels and stop overindulging in hunger.

2. Balanced Snacking:

Maintaining stable blood sugar levels is facilitated by selecting balanced snacks that include a mix of healthy fats, proteins, and carbohydrates.

Exercise and Meal Timing:

1. Pre-Exercise Meals:

Eating a healthy lunch or snack before doing out gives you the energy you need and helps keep your blood sugar stable while working out.

2. Post-Exercise Nutrition:

It's critical to time meals and snacks to coincide with exercise in order to replenish glycogen levels and promote recovery.

Considerations for Medication:

1. Coordination with Medication:

There may be precise scheduling restrictions for some diabetes medications in respect to meals. For maximum effectiveness, coordination is necessary.

Individualized Approach:

1. Personalized Meal Timing:

Given that people react differently to different meal timings, tailored strategies are essential for successful blood sugar control.

2. Regular Monitoring:

Blood sugar levels should be regularly checked before and after meals to assist people understand how differently they react to different meal times.

Challenges and Solutions:

1. Variability in Responses:

Blood sugar reactions might differ depending on a person's metabolism, the sort of food they eat, and how active they are. Frequent observation enables necessary modifications.

2. Addressing Hypoglycemia:

By maintaining a constant supply of glucose in the bloodstream, eating at the right time of day helps prevent hypoglycemia.

A key component of efficient diabetes care is knowing how timing affects blood sugar. Individuals can optimise glucose control, lower their risk of problems, and improve their general well-being by implementing strategic meal scheduling practises. It is ensured that meal timing techniques are in line with personal health goals and improve the effectiveness of diabetes treatment by regular discussion with healthcare specialists, such as dietitians and diabetes educators.

SUGGESTIONS FOR MEAL FREQUENCY

Eating at the right frequency is crucial for those with diabetes. This section offers helpful advice on meal frequency as well as tips on how to organise daily eating schedules for the best possible blood sugar control.

Regular and Balanced Meals:

1. Three Main Meals:

For the purpose of supplying necessary nutrients and regulating calorie consumption, try to have three well-balanced main meals (breakfast, lunch, and dinner).

2. Nutrient Distribution:

Evenly divide the macronutrients—fats, proteins, and carbohydrates—across the three main meals to maintain steady energy levels.

Healthy Snacks:

1. Purpose of Snacking:

Between meals, have one or two healthful snacks to help control appetite, avoid overindulging during meals, and keep blood sugar levels steady.

2. Balanced Snack Options:

Select snacks that offer a balanced food profile and long-lasting energy by combining carbohydrates with proteins or healthy fats.

Avoid Prolonged Fasting:

1. Importance of Regular Eating:

To avoid hypoglycemia (low blood sugar) and abnormal glucose patterns, avoid going extended periods without eating.

2. Consistent Meal Timing:

To control blood sugar levels and promote general metabolic health, establish a regular eating schedule.

Listen to Hunger and Fullness Cues:

1. Mindful Eating:

Observe your body's signals of hunger and fullness. To prevent overindulging, only eat when you're hungry and stop when you're full.

2. Avoiding Grazing:

While snacks are good for you, try not to graze all the time in between meals if you want to keep your eating habits consistent.

Consideration for Physical Activity:

1. Pre-Exercise Fuel:

Before beginning physical activity, have a short, well-balanced snack to give you energy without raising your blood sugar levels.

2. Post-Exercise Nutrition:

Arrange a meal or snack for after your workout to help your body recuperate and restock on glycogen.

Hydration Between Meals:

1. Role of Hydration:

Between meals, drink plenty of water to aid with digestion, reduce mindless nibbling, and preserve general health.

2. Opt for Low-Calorie Beverages:

To stay hydrated between meals without consuming extra calories or sugar, go for low-calorie liquids like water, herbal teas, or other teas.

Individualized Approach:

1. Personalized Meal Frequency:

Understand that everyone has different demands when it comes to how frequently they eat. Adjust eating habits in accordance with preferences, lifestyle, and blood sugar reactions.

2. Collaboration with Healthcare Professionals:

Together with diabetes educators and dietitians, work closely with healthcare professionals to create a customised meal schedule based on your goals and unique health requirements.

Meal frequency balancing is a dynamic process that necessitates consideration of lifestyle, blood sugar responses, and individual demands. Diabetes sufferers can develop dietary habits that support stable blood sugar levels and general well-being by include frequent, balanced meals, wholesome snacks, and being aware of their hunger cues.

ADJUSTING MEALS TO DAILY ROUTINES

Meal timing must be modified to fit everyday schedules for those with diabetes. For best blood sugar control, this section offers doable recommendations on how to coordinate meal planning with everyday routines and activities.

Morning Routine:

1. Breakfast Timing:

To boost metabolism and provide a steady blood sugar baseline for the day, aim to eat a nutritious breakfast within an hour of waking.

2. Portable Options:

For hectic mornings, think of quick and convenient breakfast options like yoghurt with berries and nuts or overnight oats.

Work or School Hours:

1. Lunch Preparation:

In order to provide sustained energy throughout the afternoon, prepare a well-balanced meal that includes lean proteins, complete grains, and an abundance of veggies.

2. Healthy Desk Snacks:

Store wholesome snacks at your workstation, like chopped veggies, fresh fruit, or almonds, to help you avoid reaching for junk food in between meals.

Afternoon Slump:

1. Smart Snacking:

Arrange a nutritious mid-afternoon snack to stave against energy slumps. For long-lasting energy, combine carbohydrates with proteins or good fats.

2. Hydration:

Avoid weariness from dehydration by staying hydrated in the afternoon. Select herbal teas or water over sugary beverages.

Evening Routine:

1. Dinner Timing:

In order to facilitate digestion and prevent any blood sugar swings during the night, try to have a well-balanced dinner at least two to three hours before going to bed.

2. Lighter Options:

For a better night's sleep and to avoid overindulging, choose lighter dinner selections.

Social and Family Gatherings:

1. Planning Ahead:

Schedule your meals around social occasions, taking into account the times of the parties and the accessibility of wholesome food options.

2. Mindful Choices:

When choosing foods for social gatherings, balance unhealthy options with indulgences.

Physical Activity:

1. Pre-Exercise Fuel:

Before beginning physical activity, have a short, well-balanced snack to give you energy without raising your blood sugar levels.

2. Post-Exercise Nutrition:

Arrange a meal or snack for after your workout to help your body recuperate and restock on glycogen.

Evening Rituals:

1. Avoiding Late-Night Snacking:

Steer clear of late-night snacks since they can cause blood sugar swings and weight gain.

2. Hydrate Before Bed:

Before going to bed, be hydrated generally by drinking water; this will not impact your blood sugar levels.

Individualized Approach:

1. Tailoring to Lifestyle:

Realise that integrating meals into everyday schedules is a customised process. Plan meals based on personal preferences, daily activities, and lifestyles.

2. Collaboration with Healthcare Professionals:

Collaborate together with diabetes educators and dietitians to develop a customised meal planning plan that meets your goals and addresses your unique health needs.

Managing diabetes properly can be achieved in a practical way by coordinating meals with daily routines. Through careful planning, thoughtful meal selection, and careful consideration of daily routines, people can establish eating habits that promote stable blood sugar levels and enhance their general well-being. Maintaining regular contact with medical experts guarantees that meal planning techniques are customised and help with diabetes control.

SNACKING STRATEGIES FOR DIABETES

When it comes to diabetes management, snacking can be crucial for people over 60. This section offers doable tactics for adding snacks to a diabetic's diet that will support general health and prevent blood sugar rises.

Healthy Snack Options:

1. Fresh Fruits:

Select fresh fruits like citrus fruits, apples, or berries. They supply vitamins and natural sweetness without significantly raising blood sugar levels.

2. Nuts and Seeds:

Choose a handful of seeds (chia seeds or pumpkin seeds) or nuts (almonds, walnuts, or pistachios) for a filling, high-nutrient snack that is high in fibre and healthy fats.

3. Greek Yogurt:

Greek yoghurt is a high-protein choice that tastes great as a balanced snack when combined with fruit or honey drizzled over it.

4. Vegetable Sticks with Hummus:

Combine bell pepper, cucumber, or carrot sticks with a dollop of hummus for a satisfyingly crunchy snack that won't send your blood sugar skyrocketing.

5. Cheese and Whole Grain Crackers:

To balance the protein and carbs and encourage fullness, pair a tiny amount of cheese with whole-grain crackers.

6. Hard-Boiled Eggs:

A quick, high-protein snack that can help you feel satisfied in between meals is hard-boiled eggs.

7. Avocado Toast:

Spread avocado on whole-grain toast for a high-nutrient snack that combines fibre, complex carbohydrates, and good fats.

Avoiding Blood Sugar Spikes:

1. Watch Portion Sizes:

Limit your portion sizes to prevent consuming too many carbohydrates, which can cause blood sugar to increase.

2. Pair Carbohydrates with Protein:

To improve blood sugar regulation and slow down the absorption of sweets, combine your carbohydrate snack with a source of protein.

3 Choose Low-Glycemic Options:

Choose low-glycemic foods to reduce the effect they have on blood sugar levels.

4. Monitor Response:

Keep a close eye on your blood sugar levels to see how various snacks impact your body's glucose reaction.

Incorporating Snacks into the Diabetic Diet:

1. Schedule Snacks Wisely:

Arrange snacks in between meals to help keep blood sugar levels consistent and prevent lengthy stretches of time without eating.

2. Integrate Snacks with Medication:

Schedule snack times in accordance with medication schedules, particularly if prescriptions call for food consumption.

3. Listen to Hunger Cues:

To avoid being overly hungry and overindulging during big meals, be aware of your hunger cues and take snacks.

4. Hydrate Alongside Snacks:

When having snacks, stay hydrated with water or other low-calorie drinks to facilitate digestion and encourage fullness.

5. Pre-Exercise Snacks:

Before beginning physical activity, have a short, well-balanced snack to give you energy without raising your blood sugar levels.

Individualized Approach:

1. Tailor Snacks to Preferences:

To guarantee enjoyment and adherence, tailor snacks according to nutritional requirements, cultural norms, and personal preferences.

2. Consult with Healthcare Professionals:

Create a customised snack plan in close collaboration with healthcare professionals, such as dietitians and diabetes educators, to meet your unique health objectives.

Snacks in the diabetes diet for those over 60 need to be carefully considered and customised for each person. Seniors with diabetes can successfully manage their condition and yet enjoy delicious, filling snacks by selecting nutrient-dense foods, preventing blood sugar rises, and including snacks into their total meal plan. Maintaining regular contact with medical professionals guarantees that snacking tactics support effective diabetes control and are in line with personal health objectives.

SPECIAL CONSIDERATIONS FOR DIABETICS

Managing diabetes entails dealing with a variety of issues that could come up because of age-related health concerns, mobility issues, and concomitant diseases. This section offers advice on how to modify the diabetic diet to suit the particular requirements of those who must take these extra precautions.

Dealing with Coexisting Conditions:

1. Understanding Comorbidities:

Be aware of the existence of concurrent medical illnesses, such as renal problems, cardiovascular diseases, or hypertension. Work together with medical specialists to develop a thorough care plan.

2. Medication Interactions:

Be aware of possible drug interactions between prescriptions for diabetes and other diseases. Effective medication management requires regular communication with healthcare providers.

3. Nutritional Strategies:

Adjust the diabetic diet to meet the unique dietary needs associated with comorbid diseases. For instance, a diet high in potassium and low in sodium may be beneficial for people with both diabetes and hypertension.

Adapting the Diet for Mobility Challenges:

1. Accessibility of Nutrient-dense Foods:

Think about how nutrient-dense foods are accessible to people who have mobility issues. To promote a balanced diet, choose options that are convenient and easily accessible.

2. Meal Preparation Assistance:

To guarantee regular compliance with dietary guidelines, look into options for meal preparation help, such as meal delivery services or the assistance of carers.

3. Convenient and Healthy Snacks:

Offer accessible, healthful snacks to cater to any mobility restrictions and encourage consistent eating habits without depending on processed or harmful foods.

Addressing Age-related Health Concerns:

1. Bone Health:

Include meals high in calcium and vitamin D to maintain bone health, which is crucial as you age. If medical specialists advise you to take supplements, do so.

2. Digestive Health:

To support digestive health and treat issues like constipation, which may be more common in older people, choose foods high in fibre.

3. Hydration:

Stress the value of maintaining adequate fluids since older people may be more susceptible to dehydration. Promote the consumption of water and include foods high in hydration, such as fruits and vegetables.

4. Regular Monitoring:

In order to proactively address age-related health risks, it is recommended to increase the frequency of health check-ups and monitoring, including frequent screenings and blood tests.

Individualized Approach:

1. Personalized Care Plans:

Collaborate with medical specialists to create individualised care plans that take into account each person's particular situation and combine the treatment of diabetes with coexisting diseases and age-related health issues.

2. Nutritional Counseling:

Consult a licenced dietitian with expertise in diabetes management for nutritional advice. They can offer individualised advice depending on a person's lifestyle, interests, and state of health.

3. Regular Communication:

Talk about any changes in your health, prescriptions, or dietary requirements with your healthcare providers in an open and consistent manner. This makes sure that the care plan is continuously modified as needed.

For diabetics, special considerations include a comprehensive approach that takes into account comorbid diseases, mobility issues, and age-related health concerns in addition to diabetes treatment. People can effectively traverse these hurdles and enhance general well-being by customising the diabetes diet to meet their unique needs, getting the right assistance, and encouraging open communication with healthcare providers.

SOCIAL AND EMOTIONAL ASPECTS OF DIET

Keeping up a healthy diet requires overcoming a variety of emotional and social obstacles. This section looks at ways that people with diabetes can manage social settings, deal with emotional difficulties, and create a network of support to improve their general well-being.

Navigating Social Situations:

1. Mindful Food Choices:

Choose your meals carefully when you go to social gatherings. Enjoy the social element of meetings while choosing healthy selections and monitoring meal amounts.

2. Communication with Hosts:

Before attending social events, let the hosts know about any dietary restrictions and make sure they are aware of any special needs for managing diabetes.

3. Bringing a Dish:

When you offer to bring something to social functions, be sure it's something healthful and fits your dietary restrictions.

4. Balancing Indulgences:

Achieve a balance between indulging in rare delicacies and staying focused on a healthy, diabetes-friendly diet.

Coping with Emotional Challenges:

1. Stress Management:

Use stress-reduction strategies to handle emotional difficulties without resorting to emotional eating, such as deep breathing, meditation, or taking up a hobby.

2. Seeking Support:

For emotional support, speak with loved ones, friends, or a mental health professional. Taking care of emotional difficulties has a positive impact on general wellbeing.

3. Journaling:

Maintain a journal as a means of self-expression and emotional release of your thoughts and feelings.

4. Identifying Triggers:

Determine the emotional factors that lead to harmful eating patterns, then focus on creating substitute coping strategies.

Building a Supportive Network:

1. Educating Loved Ones:

Encourage understanding and support by educating friends and family about diabetes and the dietary consequences of the condition.

2. Joining Support Groups:

Joining an online or in-person diabetes support group can help you connect with others going through similar things and exchange experiences.

3. Involving Loved Ones in Meal Planning:

Make meal preparation and planning a cooperative and encouraging experience by including loved ones.

4. Celebrating Achievements:

Celebrate nutritional successes and reinforce good behaviours by sharing them with your support system.

Individualized Approach:

1. Tailoring Strategies:

Understand that coping mechanisms with the social and emotional components of nutrition are quite personal. Adapt strategies to individual preferences, way of life, and emotional requirements.

2. Professional Guidance:

Seek advice from medical specialists, such as dietitians and mental health specialists, for personalised tactics that deal with particular emotional and social difficulties.

3. Regular Check-Ins:

Make an appointment for routine check-ins with your healthcare providers to talk about any emotional difficulties or dietary concerns. This guarantees continuing assistance and care plan modifications.

An essential component of diabetic management is handling the social and emotional elements of nutrition. People can improve their general well-being and successfully incorporate diabetes care into their daily life by forming a supporting network, learning effective coping methods for emotional difficulties, and navigating social settings with awareness. Frequent interaction with medical specialists guarantees that tactics support effective diabetic control and are in line with personal health objectives.

MONITORING AND ADJUSTING THE DIABETIC DIET

The flexibility to modify the diabetic diet as necessary and ongoing monitoring are essential for effective diabetes management. This section looks at the value of routine physicals, dietary modifications for better control, and progress tracking to recognise small victories along the road.

Regular Health Checkups:

1. Frequency of Checkups:

Make an appointment for routine checks with endocrinologists, nutritionists, and primary care physicians to monitor general health and evaluate the efficacy of diabetes management.

2. Blood Sugar Monitoring:

Observe a regular blood sugar monitoring regimen as prescribed by medical professionals. Frequent observation yields useful information for modifying the diabetes diet.

3. Lipid Profile and Blood Pressure Checks:

Routine health examinations should include lipid profile and blood pressure checks to address cardiovascular risk factors that are frequently linked to diabetes.

4. Comprehensive Eye Exams:

Plan thorough eye exams on a frequent basis to identify and treat any possible diabetic eye issues.

Making Adjustments for Better Control:

1. Collaborating with Healthcare Professionals:

Work together with medical specialists, such as endocrinologists and nutritionists, to analyse the findings for wellness examinations and modify the diabetic diet accordingly.

2. Medication Adjustments:

Be upfront and honest with medical professionals regarding side effects and medication adherence. Dietary concerns may be impacted by drug adjustments.

3. Assessing Carbohydrate Intake:

Analyse and modify carbohydrate consumption in response to the findings of blood sugar monitoring. Optimise the way that carbohydrates are distributed throughout the day to improve glycemic control.

4. Response to Physical Activity:

Keep an eye on how food choices affect levels of physical activity and modify meal plans as necessary to maximise energy and control blood sugar.

Tracking Progress and Celebrating Successes:

1. Keeping a Food Diary:

Keep a food journal to monitor your daily dietary decisions, which can help you see trends and determine how they affect your blood sugar levels.

2. Setting Achievable Goals:

Set attainable and reasonable nutritional objectives, such cutting back on added sugars or upping your fibre intake. Evaluate these targets' progress on a regular basis.

3. Celebrating Small Wins:

Celebrate even the smallest victories in controlling blood sugar levels or making dietary adjustments. Long-term adherence and motivation are facilitated by positive reinforcement.

4. Involving Supportive Networks:

Communicate your progress to loved ones and other supportive networks to foster a pleasant atmosphere and to promote good habits.

Individualized Approach:

1. Personalized Adjustments:

Understand that dietary modifications are quite personal. Adjust as necessary to suit individual preferences, cultural norms, and particular health objectives.

2. Regular Check-Ins:

Make time for routine check-ins with medical professionals to go over dietary modifications, track advancement, and address any issues or worries.

3. Professional Guidance:

To optimise the diabetic diet and ensure long-term success, seek professional counsel from qualified dietitians and healthcare providers.

Constant self-evaluation and cooperation with medical professionals are necessary for the continuous process of monitoring and modifying the diabetic diet. Proactive modifications, proactive health check-ups, and celebrating dietary victories are all important components of general health and successful diabetic treatment. Tailored techniques, overseen by medical experts, guarantee that dietary plans correspond with particular health requirements and objectives.

CONCLUSION

A customised diet can help manage diabetes effectively, but doing so requires a journey that includes grasping important concepts, implementing long-lasting lifestyle adjustments, and getting continuing assistance. This conclusion summarises the key nutritional concepts, offers support for long-term lifestyle modifications, and lists options for ongoing assistance.

Recap of Key Dietary Principles:

1 Individualized Meal Planning:

The significance of customised meal planning according to dietary requirements, personal preferences, and objectives for managing diabetes.

2. Balanced Nutrition:

Highlighting the need of a varied, nutrient-dense diet that is balanced in order to promote general health and wellbeing.

3. Portion Control:

The function of portion control in controlling blood sugar and avoiding excessive calorie intake.

4. Monitoring Carbohydrates:

Comprehending and overseeing the consumption of carbohydrates to enhance glycemic management.

5. Healthy Cooking Techniques:

investigating cooking methods that support heart health and maintain food's nutritional value.

6. Regular Physical Activity:

investigating cooking methods that support heart health and maintain food's nutritional value.Realising how important it is to include regular exercise in one's lifestyle in order to improve diabetes management overall.

ENCOURAGEMENT FOR SUSTAINABLE LIFESTYLE CHANGES

1. Gradual Implementation:

encouraging people to alter their eating habits gradually and sustainably so that long-term adherence is possible.

2. Positive Reinforcement:

Rewarding little victories in making healthier food choices and praising them helps to establish good habits.

3. Holistic Approach:

adopting a comprehensive strategy for managing diabetes that takes social, emotional, and lifestyle aspects into account in addition to dietary considerations.

4. Resilience in the Face of Challenges:

Inspiring resilience in the face of adversities, recognising that setbacks are a natural part of the path, and providing techniques for overcoming hurdles.

RESOURCES FOR ONGOING SUPPORT:

1. Healthcare Professionals:

Emphasising the value of continued cooperation with medical specialists, such as endocrinologists, dietitians, primary care doctors, and mental health specialists.

2. Support Groups:

Promoting the joining of online and live diabetes support groups as a way to meet people going through similar things and exchange experiences.

3. Educational Materials:

Recommending trustworthy instructional publications, websites, and other sources that offer current knowledge on food recommendations and diabetes treatment.

4. Continued Learning:

stressing the need of keeping up with the latest findings in diabetes research and therapy as well as the importance of lifelong learning about diabetes care.

In summary, the approach of controlling diabetes through nutrition is unique to each person. People with diabetes can effectively manage their condition by following important dietary guidelines, adopting lasting lifestyle adjustments, and getting continuing assistance. Despite the challenges posed by diabetes, people can live happy, healthy lives thanks to a personalised, well-balanced strategy and the encouragement of communities and healthcare providers.

MEASUREMENT CONVERSION CHART US/UK

It can be difficult to transition between U.S. & U.K. measuring units, but you can do so with ease if you have this comprehensive conversion table.

Volume Measurements:

1. Cups (Liquid):

- 1 U.S. cup = 240 milliliters
- 1 U.K. cup = 250 milliliters

2. Fluid Ounces:

- 1 U.S. fluid ounce (fl oz) = 29.57 milliliters
- 1 U.K. fluid ounce (fl oz) = 28.41 milliliters

3. Tablespoons:

- 1 U.S. tablespoon = 14.79 milliliters
- 1 U.K. tablespoon = 15 milliliters

4. Teaspoons:

- 1 U.S. teaspoon = 4.93 milliliters
- 1 U.K. teaspoon = 5 milliliters

Weight Measurements:

1. Ounces:

- 1 U.S. ounce (oz) = 28.35 grams
- 1 U.K. ounce (oz) = 28.41 grams

2. Pounds:

- 1 U.S. pound (lb) = 453.59 grams
- 1 U.K. pound (lb) = 453.59 grams

Temperature:

Temperature Conversion:

- Fahrenheit to Celsius: $°C = (°F − 32) × \frac{5}{9}$
- Celsius to Fahrenheit: $°F = (°C × \frac{9}{5}) + 32$

Notes:

- Though slight, the variations in fluid ounces and ounces between the United States and the United Kingdom can affect baking and cooking accuracy.
- Especially for important foods like baking, be sure to pay attention to whether the recipe calls for U.S. or U.K. measures.
- Make sure you're using the appropriate scale for your recipe; temperature conversions are important for oven settings.

30-DAY DIABETIC-FRIENDLY FOOD PLAN

For those with diabetes, this meal plan has been carefully designed to balance nutrition, control portion sizes, and make preparation simple. To reach a wider audience, all ingredients and nutritional information are given in both US and UK measurements. To ensure precision in the preparation of your meals, pay special attention to the details.

WEEK 1

DAY 1 (MONDAY)

1. Breakfast - Greek Yogurt Parfait

Ingredients:

- Greek yogurt (200g / 7 oz)
- Fresh berries (blueberries, strawberries) (100g / 3.5 oz)
- Chia seeds (15g / 0.5 oz)
- Almonds (chopped) (20g / 0.7 oz)
- Cinnamon (optional)

Instructions:

1. Arrange fresh berries and Greek yogurt in a bowl or glass.
2. Garnish with chopped almonds and chia seeds.
3. You can optionally add a pinch of cinnamon.

Nutritional Information (per serving):

- Calories: 250 kcal
- Protein: 15g
- Sugars: 10g

Cooking Time: No cooking time is required.

2. Lunch - Grilled Chicken Salad

Ingredients:

- Cherry tomatoes (50g / 1.8 oz)
- Chicken breast (grilled and sliced) (150g / 5.3 oz)
- Olive oil and balsamic vinegar (dressing)
- Mixed salad greens (lettuce, spinach, arugula) (100g / 3.5 oz)
- Cucumber (sliced) (50g / 1.8 oz)

Instructions:

1. Mix salad greens with grilled chicken slices.
2. Add the sliced cucumber and cherry tomatoes.
3. Toss with a dressing made of olive oil and balsamic vinegar.

Nutritional Information (per serving):

- Calories: 300 kcal
- Protein: 25g
- Sugars: 5g

Cooking Time:

- Grilling chicken: Approximately 15-20 minutes.

Please be advised that the cooking time for grilled chicken is an estimate that may change depending on the cooking method and the thickness of the chicken breast. Changes can be made in accordance with individual tastes and particular equipment.

3. Dinner - Baked Salmon with Asparagus

Ingredients:

- Asparagus spears (100g / 3.5 oz)
- Olive oil
- Salmon fillet (150g / 5.3 oz)
- Garlic (minced)
- Lemon slices

Instructions:

1. Arrange the salmon on a baking pan and preheat the oven.
2. Surround the salmon with asparagus and top with minced garlic.
3. Place lemon slices on top and drizzle with olive oil.
4. Bake the asparagus and salmon until they are soft and cooked thoroughly.

Nutritional Information (per serving):

- Calories: 300 kcal
- Protein: 30g
- Sugars: 2g

Cooking Time:

- Bake for about 15 to 20 minutes at 375°F (190°C), or until the salmon is cooked through and flakes readily when tested with a fork.

DAY 2 (TEUSDAY)

1. Breakfast - Oatmeal with Berries and Almond Milk

Ingredients:

- Almond milk (240ml / 8 fl oz)
- Oats (40g / 1.4 oz)
- Chopped almonds (15g / 0.5 oz)
- Mixed berries (blueberries, raspberries) (100g / 3.5 oz)
- Honey or sweetener (optional)

Instructions:

1. Prepare oats as directed on the packet.
2. Add almond milk, sliced almonds, and mixed berries on top.
3. If preferred, sweeten with honey or another sweetener.

Nutritional Information (per serving):

- Calories: 300 kcal
- Protein: 10g
- Sugars: 8g

2. Lunch - Quinoa Salad with Chickpeas

Ingredients:

- Chickpeas (canned, drained) (100g / 3.5 oz)
- Quinoa (cooked) (150g / 5.3 oz)
- Cherry tomatoes (50g / 1.8 oz)
- Olive oil and lemon juice (dressing)
- Feta cheese (crumbled) (30g / 1 oz)
- Cucumber (diced) (50g / 1.8 oz)

Instructions:

1. Put the cucumber, cherry tomatoes, feta cheese, chickpeas, and quinoa in a bowl.
2. For dressing, drizzle with lemon juice and olive oil.

Nutritional Information (per serving):

- Calories: 400 kcal
- Protein: 15g
- Sugars: 3g

3. Dinner - Turkey Stir-Fry with Broccoli

Ingredients:

- Olive oil
- Bell peppers (sliced) (50g / 1.8 oz)
- Turkey breast (sliced) (150g / 5.3 oz)
- Garlic and ginger (minced)
- Broccoli florets (100g / 3.5 oz)
- Soy sauce (low-sodium)

Instructions:

1. Cook turkey slices by stirring and frying them in olive oil.
2. Include the bell peppers, broccoli, ginger, and garlic.
3. Cook the vegetables until they are soft and drizzle with soy sauce.

Nutritional Information (per serving):

- Calories: 350 kcal
- Protein: 30g
- Sugars: 5g

4. Snack - Apple Slices with Peanut Butter

Ingredients:

- Apple (sliced) (1 medium)
- Peanut butter (natural, no added sugar) (15g / 0.5 oz)

Instructions:

1. Cut the apple into slices and coat each piece with peanut butter.

Nutritional Information (per serving):

- Calories: 150 kcal
- Protein: 3g
- Sugars: 10g

ADDITIONAL SNACK OPTIONS

1. Cottage Cheese with Pineapple

Ingredients:

- Cottage cheese (low-fat) (150g / 5.3 oz)
- Pineapple chunks (100g / 3.5 oz)

Instructions:

1. Mix cottage cheese with pineapple chunks.

Nutritional Information (per serving):

- Calories: 200 kcal
- Protein: 15g
- Sugars: 10g

2. Stuffed Bell Peppers with Turkey and Quinoa

Ingredients:

- Mozzarella cheese (shredded) (30g / 1 oz)
- Bell peppers (halved and cleaned) (2 medium)
- Quinoa (cooked) (100g / 3.5 oz)
- Tomato sauce (low-sugar) (200ml / 6.8 fl oz)
- Turkey (cooked and ground) (150g / 5.3 oz)

Instructions:

1. Set the oven to preheat. Combine the quinoa, tomato sauce, and cooked turkey in a bowl.
2. Stuff mixture into bell peppers and replace tops with mozzarella.
3. Bake for the cheese to melt and the peppers to become soft.

Nutritional Information (per serving):

- Calories: 300 kcal
- Protein: 20g
- Sugars: 5g

DAY 3 (WEDNESDAY)

1. Breakfast - Spinach and Feta Omelet

Ingredients:

- Spinach (fresh, chopped) (50g / 1.8 oz)
- Eggs (2 large)
- Feta cheese (crumbled) (30g / 1 oz)
- Salt and pepper to taste
- Olive oil

Instructions:

1. Whisk the eggs in a bowl and add pepper and salt to taste.
2. Add the spinach to a pan with heated olive oil and simmer until wilted.
3. Cover the spinach with whisked eggs, top with feta, and simmer until set.

Nutritional Information (per serving):

- Calories: 300 kcal
- Protein: 20g
- Sugars: 2g

Cooking Time: 10 minutes

2. Lunch - Black Bean and Vegetable Wrap

Ingredients:

- Black beans (canned, drained) (100g / 3.5 oz)
- Mixed vegetables (bell peppers, onions, tomatoes) (150g / 5.3 oz)
- Whole-grain wrap
- Greek yogurt (plain, for dressing)

Instructions:

1. Reheat the mixed vegetables & black beans.
2. Spoon the mixture into a whole-grain wrapper.
3. For the dressing, drizzle on some plain Greek yogurt.

Nutritional Information (per serving):

- Calories: 350 kcal
- Protein: 15g
- Sugars: Approximately 5g

Cooking Time: 15 minutes

3 Dinner - Baked Cod with Lemon and Herbs

Ingredients:

- Fresh herbs (parsley, dill)
- Cod fillet (150g / 5.3 oz)
- Garlic (minced)
- Lemon (sliced)
- Olive oil

Instructions:
1. Arrange the fish on a baking sheet and preheat the oven.
2. Add minced garlic, fresh herbs, and lemon slices on top.
3. Drizzle with olive oil, then bake the fish for the desired amount of doneness.

Nutritional Information (per serving):

- Calories: 250 kcal
- Protein: 25g
- Sugars: 1g

Cooking Time: 20 minutes

4 Snack - Yogurt and Berry Smoothie

Ingredients:

- Almond milk (unsweetened) (200ml / 6.8 fl oz)
- Mixed berries (strawberries, blueberries) (100g / 3.5 oz)
- Greek yogurt (unsweetened) (150g / 5.3 oz)
- Chia seeds (optional)

Instructions:
1. Blend the almond milk, chia seeds, Greek yogurt, and mixed berries until smooth.

Nutritional Information (per serving):

- Calories: 200 kcal
- Protein: 10g
- Sugars: 8g

Preparation Time: 5 minutes

ADDITIONAL SNACK OPTIONS

1. Edamame Beans

Ingredients:

- Edamame beans (steamed) (150g / 5.3 oz)
- Sea salt (to taste)

Instructions:
1. Add sea salt and steam the edamame beans.

Nutritional Information (per serving):

- Calories: 150 kcal
- Protein: 12g
- Sugars: 2g

Cooking Time: 5 minutes

2. Salmon and Avocado Sushi Rolls

Ingredients:

- Avocado (sliced)
- Brown rice (cooked)
- Nori seaweed sheets
- Soy sauce (low-sodium)
- Cooked salmon (flaked) (150g / 5.3 oz)

Instructions:

1. Take a bamboo sushi mat and place a sheet of nori seaweed on it.
2. Place avocado, salmon, and brown rice on the nori.
3. Slicing into sushi rolls, roll tightly. Accompany with soy sauce reduced in sodium.

Nutritional Information (per serving):

- Calories: 300 kcal
- Protein: 15g
- Sugars: 2g

Cooking Time: 30 minutes (assuming rice is pre-cooked)

DAY 4 (THURSDAY)

1. Breakfast - Whole Grain Toast with Avocado and Tomato

Ingredients:

- Avocado (mashed) (1/2)
- Whole grain bread (2 slices)
- Tomato (sliced)
- Salt and pepper to taste

Instructions:

1. Toast the slices of whole grain bread.
2. Top the toast with sliced tomato after spreading mashed avocado over it.
3. Add salt and pepper to taste.

Nutritional Information (per serving):

- Calories: 250 kcal
- Protein: 8g
- Sugars: 3g

Cooking Time: 10 minutes

2. Lunch - Shrimp and Vegetable Stir-Fry

Ingredients:

- Ginger and garlic (minced)
- Shrimp (peeled and deveined) (150g / 5.3 oz)
- Mixed vegetables (broccoli, bell peppers, snow peas) (150g / 5.3 oz)
- Sesame oil

- Soy sauce (low-sodium)

Instructions:

1. Add garlic and ginger to sesame oil and stir-fry prawns.
2. Cook the mixed veggies until they are soft by adding soy sauce.

Nutritional Information (per serving):

- Calories: 300 kcal
- Protein: 20g
- Sugars: 4g

Cooking Time: 15 minutes

3. Dinner - Eggplant and Chickpea Curry

Ingredients:

- Chickpeas (canned, drained) (150g / 5.3 oz)
- Onion and tomatoes (diced)
- Eggplant (cubed) (200g / 7 oz)
- Coconut milk (light)
- Curry spices (turmeric, cumin, coriander)

Instructions:

1. In a pan, sauté the eggplant, tomatoes, and onion.
2. Stir in coconut milk, curry powder, and chickpeas. Simmer the aubergine until it becomes soft.

Nutritional Information (per serving):

- Calories: 350 kcal
- Protein: 15g
- Sugars: 5g
- Cooking Time: 25 minutes

4. Snack - Mixed Nuts

Ingredients:

- Mixed nuts (almonds, walnuts, pistachios) (30g / 1 oz)

Instructions:

1. Combine and savor a few pieces of mixed nuts.

Nutritional Information (per serving):

- Calories: 200 kcal
- Protein: 5g
- Sugars: 1g

ADDITIONAL SNACK OPTIONS

1. Roasted Chickpeas

Ingredients:

- Paprika and cumin (seasoning)

- Chickpeas (canned, drained) (150g / 5.3 oz)
- Olive oil

Instructions:

1. Toss chickpeas with spices and olive oil.
2. Roast till crispy in the oven.

Nutritional Information (per serving):

- Calories: 150 kcal
- Protein: 6g
- Sugars: 2g

Cooking Time: 20 minutes

2. Mushroom and Spinach Stuffed Chicken Breast

Ingredients:

- Garlic powder and Italian seasoning
- Mushrooms and spinach (sautéed)
- Olive oil
- Chicken breast (boneless and skinless) (150g / 5.3 oz)

Instructions:

1. Make a pocket in the chicken breast and insert the spinach and sautéed mushrooms inside.
2. Add some Italian seasoning and garlic powder to your food.
3. Continue baking the chicken until it's fully done.

Nutritional Information (per serving):

- Calories: 300 kcal
- Protein: 25g
- Sugars: 3g

Cooking Time: 30 minutes (assuming sautéed ingredients are pre-cooked)

DAY 5 (FRIDAY)

1. Breakfast - Scrambled Eggs With Spinach And Tomatoes

Ingredients:

- 2 large eggs
- 1 cup fresh spinach
- 1/2 cup cherry tomatoes
- 1 tsp olive oil

Instructions

1. Cook eggs with spinach and tomatoes in olive oil. Season with herbs.

Nutritional Information:

- Calories: 250
- Protein: 18g
- Sugar: 2g

Cooking Time: 10 minutes

2. Lunch: Meal - Grilled Chicken Salad With Mixed Greens

Ingredients:

- 4 oz grilled chicken breast
- 2 cups mixed salad greens
- 1/2 cucumber, sliced
- 2 tbsp vinaigrette dressing (olive oil and vinegar)

Instructions:

1. Grill chicken breast and toss with mixed greens, cucumber, and a vinaigrette dressing.

Nutritional Information:

- Calories: 300
- Protein: 25g
- Sugar: 4g

Cooking Time: 15 minutes

3. Snack - Greek Yogurt With Berries

Ingredients:

- 1/2 cup plain Greek yogurt
- 1/2 cup mixed berries

Instructions:

1. Mix plain Greek yogurt with fresh berries.

Nutritional Information:

- Calories: 150
- Protein: 15g
- Sugar: 10g

4. Dinner - Baked Salmon With Quinoa And Steamed Broccoli

Ingredients:

- 6 oz salmon fillet
- 1/2 cup quinoa (cooked)
- 1 cup broccoli, steamed

Instructions:

1. Bake salmon, serve over cooked quinoa, and steamed broccoli on the side.

Nutritional Information:

- Calories: 400
- Protein: 30g
- Sugar: 2g

Cooking Time: 25 minutes

DAY 6 (SATURDAY)

1. Breakfast - Overnight Oats With Almond Milk, Chia Seeds, And Berries

Ingredients:

- 1/2 cup rolled oats
- 1 cup unsweetened almond milk
- 1 tbsp chia seeds
- 1/2 cup mixed berries

Instructions:

1. Combine oats, almond milk, chia seeds, and refrigerate overnight.
2. Top with berries in the morning.

Nutritional Information:

- Calories: 280
- Protein: 10g
- Sugar: 8g

Preparation Time: 5 minutes (plus overnight refrigeration)

2. Lunch: Quinoa And Black Bean Bowl With Avocado

Ingredients:

- 1/2 cup quinoa (cooked)
- 1/2 cup black beans (canned, rinsed)
- 1/2 avocado, diced

Instructions:

1. Mix cooked quinoa and black beans, top with diced avocado.

Nutritional Information:

- Calories: 350
- Protein: 15g
- Sugar: 3g

Preparation Time: 20 minutes

3. Snack: Sliced Cucumber With Hummus

Ingredients:

- 1 medium cucumber, sliced
- 2 tbsp hummus

Instructions:

1. Slice cucumber and serve with hummus.

Nutritional Information:

- Calories: 100
- Protein: 4g

- Sugar: 2g

4. Dinner - Stir-Fried Tofu With Broccoli And Brown Rice

Ingredients:

- 8 oz tofu, cubed
- 1 cup broccoli florets
- 1 cup brown rice (cooked)

Instructions:

1. Stir-fry tofu with broccoli in olive oil, serve over cooked brown rice.

Nutritional Information:

- Calories: 380
- Protein: 20g
- Sugar: 2g

Cooking Time: 15 minutes

DAY 7 (SUNDAY)

1. Breakfast - Whole Grain Toast With Mashed Avocado And Poached Egg

Ingredients:

- 2 slices whole grain bread
- 1/2 avocado, mashed
- 1 poached egg

Instructions:

1. Toast whole grain bread, spread mashed avocado
2. Top with a poached egg.

Nutritional Information:

- Calories: 300
- Protein: 15g
- Sugar: 2g

Cooking Time: 10 minutes

2. Lunch - Turkey And Vegetable Wrap With Whole Wheat Tortilla

Ingredients:

- 4 oz sliced turkey breast
- 1 whole wheat tortilla
- Lettuce, tomato, cucumber slices

Instructions:

1. Fill a whole wheat tortilla with sliced turkey, lettuce, tomato, and cucumber.

Nutritional Information:

- Calories: 320
- Protein: 25g
- Sugar: 4g

3. Snack: Handful of mixed nuts

Ingredients:

- Almonds, walnuts, pistachios, etc.

Nutritional Information:

- Calories: 200
- Protein: 7g
- Sugar: 1g

4. Dinner: Grilled Shrimp With Quinoa And Roasted Vegetables

Ingredients:

- 6 oz shrimp, peeled and deveined
- 1 cup quinoa (cooked)
- Mixed roasted vegetables (bell peppers, zucchini, cherry tomatoes)

Instructions:

1. Grill shrimp, serve over cooked quinoa, and roasted vegetables.

Nutritional Information:

- Calories: 400
- Protein: 30g
- Sugar: 3g

Cooking Time: 20 minutes

WEEK 2

DAY 8 (MONDAY)

Breakfast: Greek Yogurt Parfait With Granola And Berries

Ingredients:

- 1 cup Greek yogurt
- 1/2 cup granola
- 1/2 cup mixed berries

Instructions:

1. Layer Greek yogurt with granola and mixed berries.

Nutritional Information:

- Calories: 320
- Protein: 15g
- Sugar: 10g

2. Lunch: Lentil soup with a side of mixed greens

Ingredients:

- 1 cup lentil soup (homemade or low-sodium canned)
- 2 cups mixed salad greens
- 1 tbsp olive oil for dressing

Instructions:

1. Prepare lentil soup, serve with a side of mixed green salad.

Nutritional Information:

- Calories: 350
- Protein: 18g
- Sugar: 5g

Cooking Time: 30 minutes

3. Snack: Apple slices with almond butter

Ingredients:

- 1 medium apple, sliced
- 2 tbsp almond butter

Instructions:

1. Slice apple and dip in almond butter.

Nutritional Information:

- Calories: 200
- Protein: 5g
- Sugar: 10g

4. Dinner: Baked Chicken Breast With Sweet Potato And Steamed Broccoli

Ingredients:

- 6 oz chicken breast
- 1 medium sweet potato, cubed
- 1 cup broccoli, steamed

Instructions:

1. Bake chicken breast, serve with roasted sweet potato and steamed broccoli.

Nutritional Information:

- Calories: 450
- Protein: 35g
- Sugar: 5g

Cooking Time: 30 minutes

DAY 9 (TEUSDAY)

1. Breakfast: Smoothie With Spinach, Banana, And Almond Milk

Ingredients:

- 1 cup fresh spinach
- 1 banana
- 1 cup unsweetened almond milk

Instructions:

1. Blend spinach, banana, and almond milk until smooth.

Nutritional Information:

- Calories: 200
- Protein: 5g
- Sugar: 12g

2. Lunch: Turkey And Vegetable Kebabs With Quinoa

Ingredients:

- 4 oz turkey breast, cubed
- Assorted vegetables (bell peppers, cherry tomatoes, zucchini)
- 1/2 cup quinoa (cooked)

Instructions:

1. Skewer turkey cubes and vegetables
2. Grill, and serve with a side of quinoa.

Nutritional Information:

- Calories: 350
- Protein: 25g

- Sugar: 4g

Cooking Time: 15 minutes

3. Snack: Hummus-stuffed bell peppers

Ingredients:

- 2 bell peppers, sliced
- 4 tbsp hummus

Instructions:

1. Cut bell peppers into strips and fill with hummus.

Nutritional Information:

- Calories: 120
- Protein: 4g
- Sugar: 3g

4. Dinner: Grilled salmon with quinoa and steamed asparagus

Ingredients:

- 6 oz salmon fillet
- 1/2 cup quinoa (cooked)
- 1 cup asparagus, steamed

Instructions:

1. Grill salmon, serve with quinoa, and steamed asparagus on the side.

Nutritional Information:

- Calories: 420
- Protein: 30g
- Sugar: 3g

Cooking Time: 25 minutes

DAY 10 (WEDNESDAY)

1. Breakfast: Chia seed pudding with almond milk and berries

Ingredients:

- 2 tbsp chia seeds
- 1 cup unsweetened almond milk
- 1/2 cup mixed berries

Instructions:

1. Mix chia seeds with almond milk
2. Refrigerate overnight, and top with fresh berries.

Nutritional Information:

- Calories: 250
- Protein: 7g
- Sugar: 6g

Preparation Time: 5 minutes (plus overnight refrigeration)

2. Lunch: Shrimp and avocado salad with mixed greens

Ingredients:

- 6 oz shrimp, peeled and deveined
- 2 cups mixed salad greens
- 1/2 avocado, sliced
- Cherry tomatoes

Instructions:

1. Sauté shrimp and toss with mixed greens, cherry tomatoes, and sliced avocado.

Nutritional Information:

- Calories: 300
- Protein: 20g
- Sugar: 5g

Cooking Time: 15 minutes

3. Snack: Cottage cheese with sliced peaches

Ingredients:

- 1/2 cup low-fat cottage cheese
- 1 peach, sliced

Instructions:

1. Combine cottage cheese with fresh sliced peaches.

Nutritional Information:

- Calories: 150
- Protein: 12g
- Sugar: 8g

4. Dinner: Baked chicken thighs with sweet potato and green beans

Ingredients:

- 6 oz chicken thighs
- 1 medium sweet potato, cubed
- 1 cup green beans, steamed

Instructions:

1. Bake chicken thighs, serve with roasted sweet potatoes, and steamed green beans.

Nutritional Information:

- Calories: 450

- Protein: 30g
- Sugar: 6g

Cooking Time: 35 minutes

DAY 11 (THURSDAY)

1. Breakfast: Omelette with spinach, feta cheese, and whole-grain toast

Ingredients:

- 3 large eggs
- 1 cup fresh spinach
- 2 tbsp feta cheese
- 2 slices whole-grain bread

Instructions:

1. Whisk eggs, sauté spinach, and feta
2. Then pour over eggs. Serve with whole-grain toast.

Nutritional Information:

- Calories: 350
- Protein: 20g
- Sugar: 2g

Cooking Time: 15 minutes

2. Lunch: Quinoa and black bean power bowl with salsa

Ingredients:

- 1 cup quinoa (cooked)
- 1/2 cup black beans (canned, rinsed)
- Corn kernels
- 1/4 cup salsa

Instructions:

1. Mix quinoa, black beans, corn, and top with salsa.

Nutritional Information:

- Calories: 380
- Protein: 15g
- Sugar: 5g

3. Snack: Apple slices with almond butter

Ingredients:

- 1 medium apple, sliced
- 2 tbsp almond butter

Nutritional Information:

- Calories: 200

- Protein: 5g
- Sugar: 10g

4. Dinner: Baked chicken breast with sweet potato and green beans

Ingredients:

- 6 oz chicken breast
- 1 medium sweet potato, cubed
- 1 cup green beans, steamed

Instructions:

1. Bake chicken breast, serve with roasted sweet potatoes
2. Steamed green beans.

Nutritional Information:

- Calories: 450
- Protein: 30g
- Sugar: 6g

Cooking Time: 30 minutes

DAY 12 (FRIDAY)

1. Breakfast: Greek yogurt parfait with granola and mixed berries

Ingredients:

- 1 cup Greek yogurt
- 1/2 cup granola
- 1/2 cup mixed berries

Instructions:

1. Layer Greek yogurt with granola and a mix of berries.

Nutritional Information:

- Calories: 320
- Protein: 15g
- Sugar: 10g

2. Lunch: Turkey and avocado wrap with whole wheat tortilla

Ingredients:

- 4 oz sliced turkey breast
- 1 whole wheat tortilla
- 1/2 avocado, sliced
- Lettuce, tomato

Instructions:

1. Fill a whole wheat tortilla with sliced turkey, avocado, lettuce, and tomato.

Nutritional Information:

- Calories: 350
- Protein: 25g
- Sugar: 4g

3. Snack: Carrot and cucumber sticks with hummus

Ingredients:

- 1 cup carrot sticks
- 1 cup cucumber sticks
- 4 tbsp hummus

Nutritional Information:

- Calories: 150
- Protein: 5g
- Sugar: 4g

4. Dinner: Grilled salmon with quinoa and sautéed asparagus

Ingredients:

- 6 oz salmon fillet
- 1/2 cup quinoa (cooked)
- 1 cup asparagus, sautéed

Instructions:

1. Grill salmon, serve with quinoa, and asparagus sautéed in olive oil.

Nutritional Information:

- Calories: 420
- Protein: 30g
- Sugar: 3g

Cooking Time: 25 minutes

DAY 13 (SATURDAY)

1. Breakfast: Smoothie with kale, banana, and almond milk

Ingredients:

- 1 cup fresh kale
- 1 banana
- 1 cup unsweetened almond milk

Instructions:

1. Blend kale, banana, and almond milk until smooth.

Nutritional Information:

- Calories: 200
- Protein: 7g
- Sugar: 8g

2. Lunch: Chickpea salad with tomatoes, cucumbers, and feta cheese
Ingredients:

- 1 cup canned chickpeas (rinsed)
- 1 cup cherry tomatoes, halved
- 1/2 cucumber, diced
- 2 tbsp crumbled feta cheese

Instructions:

1. Toss chickpeas with diced tomatoes, cucumbers, and crumbled feta cheese.

Nutritional Information:

- Calories: 320
- Protein: 14g
- Sugar: 6g

3. Snack: Handful of mixed nuts
Ingredients:

- Almonds, walnuts, pistachios, etc.

Nutritional Information:

- Calories: 200
- Protein: 7g
- Sugar: 1g

4. Dinner: Stir-fried tofu with broccoli and brown rice
Ingredients:

- 8 oz tofu, cubed
- 1 cup broccoli florets
- 1 cup brown rice (cooked)

Instructions:

1. Stir-fry tofu with broccoli in olive oil, serve over cooked brown rice.

Nutritional Information:

- Calories: 380
- Protein: 20g
- Sugar: 2g

Cooking Time: 20 minutes

DAY 14 (SUNDAY)
1. Breakfast: Whole grain toast with smoked salmon and cream cheese
Ingredients:

- 2 slices whole grain bread
- 2 oz smoked salmon

- 2 tbsp cream cheese

Instructions:

1. Toast whole grain bread, spread cream cheese, and top with smoked salmon.

Nutritional Information:

- Calories: 300
- Protein: 18g
- Sugar: 2g

2. Lunch: Lentil soup with a side of mixed greens

Ingredients:

- 1 cup lentil soup (homemade or low-sodium canned)
- 2 cups mixed salad greens
- 1 tbsp olive oil for dressing

Nutritional Information:

- Calories: 350
- Protein: 18g
- Sugar: 5g

Cooking Time: 30 minutes

3. Snack: Meal: Banana with almond butter

Ingredients:

- 1 medium banana
- 2 tbsp almond butter

Nutritional Information:

- Calories: 220
- Protein: 5g
- Sugar: 10g

4. Dinner: Baked cod with quinoa and roasted Brussels sprouts

Ingredients:

- 6 oz cod fillet
- 1/2 cup quinoa (cooked)
- 1 cup Brussels sprouts, halved

Instructions:

1. Bake cod, serve with quinoa, and roasted Brussels sprouts.

Nutritional Information:

- Calories: 400
- Protein: 30g

- Sugar: 3g

Cooking Time: 25 minutes

WEEK 3

DAY 15 (MONDAY)

1. Breakfast: Overnight oats with almond milk, sliced almonds, and banana

Ingredients:

- 1/2 cup rolled oats
- 1 cup unsweetened almond milk
- 2 tbsp sliced almonds
- 1 banana, sliced

Instructions:

Combine oats, almond milk, sliced almonds, and banana slices. Refrigerate overnight.

Nutritional Information:

- Calories: 300
- Protein: 10g
- Sugar: 8g

Preparation Time: 5 minutes (plus overnight refrigeration)

2. Lunch: Caprese salad with grilled chicken

Ingredients:

- 4 oz grilled chicken breast
- Tomato slices
- Fresh mozzarella slices
- Fresh basil leaves
- Balsamic glaze

Instructions:

1. Combine tomato slices, fresh mozzarella, basil, and grilled chicken.
2. Drizzle with balsamic glaze.

Nutritional Information:

- Calories: 350
- Protein: 25g
- Sugar: 5g

3. Snack: Greek yogurt with honey and walnuts

Ingredients:

- 1 cup plain Greek yogurt
- 1 tbsp honey
- 2 tbsp chopped walnuts

Nutritional Information:

- Calories: 250
- Protein: 15g
- Sugar: 12g

4. Dinner: Turkey and vegetable stir-fry with brown rice

Ingredients:

- 8 oz lean ground turkey
- Mixed vegetables (broccoli, snap peas, carrots)
- 1 cup brown rice (cooked)

Instructions:

1. Stir-fry lean ground turkey with a mix of vegetables and serve over brown rice.

Nutritional Information:

- Calories: 400
- Protein: 26g
- Sugar: 4g

Cooking Time: 20 minutes

DAY 16 (TEUSDAY)

1. Breakfast: Banana and blueberry smoothie with spinach

Ingredients:

- 1 banana
- 1/2 cup blueberries
- Handful of fresh spinach
- 1 cup unsweetened almond milk

Instructions:

1. Blend banana, blueberries, spinach, and almond milk until smooth.

Nutritional Information:

- Calories: 250
- Protein: 7g
- Sugar: 14g

2. Lunch: Quinoa and vegetable-stuffed bell peppers

Ingredients:

- 1 cup quinoa (cooked)
- Mixed vegetables (zucchini, corn, tomatoes)
- 4 bell peppers, halved

Instructions:

1. Mix cooked quinoa with a variety of vegetables, stuff bell peppers, and bake.

Nutritional Information:

- Calories: 350
- Protein: 15g
- Sugar: 6g

Cooking Time: 30 minutes

3. Snack: Edamame with sea salt

Ingredients:

- 1 cup edamame (boiled)
- Sea salt to taste

Instructions:

1. Boil edamame and sprinkle with sea salt.

Nutritional Information:

- Calories: 150
- Protein: 14g
- Sugar: 3g

4. Dinner: Shrimp and vegetable skewers with quinoa

Ingredients:

- 8 oz shrimp, peeled and deveined
- Mixed vegetables (bell peppers, cherry tomatoes, red onion)
- 1 cup quinoa (cooked)

Instructions:

1. Skewer shrimp and a variety of vegetables, grill, and serve with quinoa.

Nutritional Information:

- Calories: 380
- Protein: 30g
- Sugar: 3g

Cooking Time: 20 minutes

DAY 17 (WEDNESDAY)

1. Breakfast: Avocado toast with poached egg and cherry tomatoes

Ingredients:

- 1 slice whole-grain bread
- 1/2 avocado, mashed
- 1 poached egg
- Cherry tomatoes, halved

Instructions:

1. Mash avocado on whole-grain toast, top with a poached egg and cherry tomatoes.

Nutritional Information:

- Calories: 300
- Protein: 15g
- Sugar: 3g

Cooking Time: 15 minutes

2. Lunch: *Whole grain wrap with grilled vegetables and hummus*

Ingredients:

- Mixed grilled vegetables (zucchini, bell peppers, eggplant)
- 1 whole grain tortilla
- 2 tbsp hummus

Instructions:

1. Grill a mix of vegetables, wrap in a whole-grain tortilla, and spread with hummus.

Nutritional Information:

- Calories: 350
- Protein: 12g
- Sugar: 5g

3. Snack: *Cottage cheese with sliced strawberries*

Ingredients:

- 1/2 cup low-fat cottage cheese
- 1/2 cup sliced strawberries

Nutritional Information:

- Calories: 150
- Protein: 12g
- Sugar: 8g

4. Dinner: *Baked chicken thighs with quinoa and roasted sweet potatoes*

Ingredients:

- 6 oz chicken thighs
- 1 cup quinoa (cooked)
- 1 medium sweet potato, cubed

Instructions:

1. Bake chicken thighs, serve with quinoa, and roasted sweet potatoes.

Nutritional Information:

- Calories: 450
- Protein: 30g
- Sugar: 6g

Cooking Time: 35 minutes

DAY 18 (THURSDAY)

1. Breakfast: Berry and Spinach Smoothie Bowl

Ingredients:

- 1 cup mixed berries (strawberries, blueberries, raspberries)
- Handful of fresh spinach
- 1/2 cup Greek yogurt
- 1/4 cup unsweetened almond milk
- 1 tbsp sliced almonds
- 1 tbsp chia seeds

Instructions:

1. Blend mixed berries, spinach, Greek yogurt, and a splash of almond milk.
2. Top with sliced almonds and chia seeds.

Nutritional Information:

- Calories: 300
- Protein: 15g
- Sugar: 12g

2. Lunch: Quinoa Salad with Chickpeas and Mediterranean Veggies

Ingredients:

- 1 cup quinoa (cooked)
- 1/2 cup canned chickpeas (rinsed)
- Cherry tomatoes, halved
- 1/2 cucumber, diced
- Kalamata olives, sliced
- Feta cheese, crumbled
- Olive oil and lemon juice for dressing

Instructions:

- Toss cooked quinoa with chickpeas, cherry tomatoes, cucumber, olives, and feta cheese.
- Drizzle with olive oil and lemon juice.

Nutritional Information:

- Calories: 380
- Protein: 18g
- Sugar: 5g

3. Snack: Greek Yogurt with Honey and Pistachios

Ingredients:

- 1 cup plain Greek yogurt
- 1 tbsp honey

- 2 tbsp chopped pistachios

Nutritional Information:

- Calories: 250
- Protein: 15g
- Sugar: 10g

4. Dinner: Stir-Fried Tofu with Broccoli and Brown Rice

Ingredients:

- 8 oz tofu, cubed
- 1 cup broccoli florets
- Mixed vegetables (bell peppers, snap peas)
- 1 cup brown rice (cooked)
- Soy sauce for seasoning

Instructions:

- Sauté tofu, broccoli, and other veggies in a light soy sauce.
- Serve over cooked brown rice.

Nutritional Information:

- Calories: 400
- Protein: 20g
- Sugar: 2g

Cooking Time: 20 minutes

DAY 19 (FRIDAY)

1. Breakfast: Avocado and Tomato Toast with Poached Egg

Ingredients:

- 1 slice whole-grain bread
- 1/2 avocado, mashed
- 1 medium tomato, sliced
- 1 poached egg

Instructions:

1. Mash avocado on whole-grain toast, top with sliced tomatoes, and a poached egg.

Nutritional Information:

- Calories: 320
- Protein: 15g
- Sugar: 3g

Cooking Time: 15 minutes

2. Lunch: Spinach and Feta Stuffed Chicken Breast

Ingredients:

- 6 oz chicken breast
- Handful of fresh spinach
- 2 tbsp feta cheese
- Olive oil for brushing

Instructions:

1. Butterfly chicken breast, stuff with spinach and feta, and bake until cooked through.

Nutritional Information:

- Calories: 350
- Protein: 30g
- Sugar: 2g

Cooking Time: 30 minutes

3. Snack: Apple Slices with Almond Butter

Ingredients:

- 1 medium apple, sliced
- 2 tbsp almond butter

Nutritional Information:

- Calories: 200
- Protein: 5g
- Sugar: 10g

1. Dinner: Shrimp and Vegetable Stir-Fry with Quinoa

Ingredients:

- 8 oz shrimp, peeled and deveined
- Mixed vegetables (bell peppers, snap peas, carrots)
- 1 cup quinoa (cooked)
- Teriyaki sauce for seasoning

Instructions:

1. Stir-fry shrimp, mixed vegetables, and serve over quinoa with a light teriyaki sauce.

Nutritional Information:

- Calories: 380
- Protein: 30g
- Sugar: 4g

Cooking Time: 20 minutes

DAY 20 (SATURDAY)

1. Breakfast: Peanut Butter Banana Overnight Oats

Ingredients:

- 1/2 cup rolled oats
- 1 cup unsweetened almond milk
- 2 tbsp peanut butter
- 1 banana, sliced

Instructions:

1. Mix rolled oats, almond milk, peanut butter, and sliced bananas.
2. Refrigerate overnight.

Nutritional Information:

- Calories: 300
- Protein: 10g
- Sugar: 8g

Preparation Time: 5 minutes (plus overnight refrigeration)

2. Lunch: Turkey and Quinoa Stuffed Bell Peppers

Ingredients:

- 8 oz lean ground turkey
- 1 cup quinoa (cooked)
- 4 bell peppers, halved

Instructions:

1. Mix cooked quinoa with lean ground turkey, stuff bell peppers, and bake.

Nutritional Information:

- Calories: 400
- Protein: 26g
- Sugar: 5g

Cooking Time: 30 minutes

3. Snack: Carrot and Hummus Snack Box

Ingredients:

- 1 cup carrot sticks
- 4 tbsp hummus

Nutritional Information:

- Calories: 150
- Protein: 5g
- Sugar: 4g

4. Dinner: Grilled Salmon with Quinoa and Steamed Asparagus

Ingredients:

- 6 oz salmon fillet
- 1/2 cup quinoa (cooked)
- 1 cup asparagus, steamed

Instructions:

1. Grill salmon, serve with quinoa, and steamed asparagus on the side.

Nutritional Information:

- Calories: 420
- Protein: 30g
- Sugar: 3g

Cooking Time: 25 minutes

DAY 21 (SUNDAY)

1. Breakfast: Blueberry and Almond Butter Smoothie

Ingredients:

- 1 cup blueberries
- 2 tbsp almond butter
- 1/2 cup Greek yogurt
- 1 cup unsweetened almond milk

Instructions:

1. Blend blueberries, almond butter, Greek yogurt, and almond milk until smooth.

Nutritional Information:

- Calories: 250
- Protein: 10g
- Sugar: 12g

2. Lunch: Lentil and Vegetable Soup with a Side Salad

Ingredients:

- 1 cup lentil and vegetable soup (homemade or low-sodium canned)
- 2 cups mixed salad greens
- 1 tbsp olive oil for dressing

Instructions:

1. Prepare lentil and vegetable soup and serve with a side salad.

Nutritional Information:

- Calories: 350
- Protein: 18g
- Sugar: 5g

Cooking Time: 30 minutes

3. Snack: Banana and Walnut Muffins (2 pieces)

Ingredients:

- 2 medium-sized banana and walnut muffins (prepared with whole wheat flour and minimal sugar)

Nutritional Information:

- Calories: 200
- Protein: 5g
- Sugar: 8g

4. Dinner: Baked Cod with Quinoa and Roasted Brussels Sprouts

Ingredients:

- 6 oz cod fillet
- 1/2 cup quinoa (cooked)
- 1 cup Brussels sprouts, halved

Instructions:

1. Bake cod, serve with quinoa, and roasted Brussels sprouts.

Nutritional Information:

- Calories: 400
- Protein: 30g
- Sugar: 3g

Cooking Time: 25 minutes

WEEK 4

DAY 22 (MONDAY)

1. Breakfast: Whole Grain Pancakes with Mixed Berries

Ingredients:

- 2 whole grain pancakes
- 1/2 cup mixed berries (strawberries, blueberries, raspberries)

Instructions:

1. Prepare whole grain pancakes and top with a mix of fresh berries.

Nutritional Information:

- Calories: 350
- Protein: 10g
- Sugar: 10g

Cooking Time: 15 minutes

2. Lunch: Chickpea and Avocado Wrap

Ingredients:

- 1 whole wheat tortilla
- 1/2 cup mashed chickpeas
- 1/2 avocado, sliced
- Cherry tomatoes, halved
- Lettuce

Instructions:

1. Fill a whole wheat wrap with mashed chickpeas, sliced avocado, cherry tomatoes, and lettuce.

Nutritional Information:

- Calories: 350
- Protein: 15g
- Sugar: 4g

3. Snack: Trail Mix with Dried Fruits and Nuts

Ingredients:

- Almonds, walnuts, pistachios, dried cranberries, and dried apricots

Nutritional Information:

- Calories: 200
- Protein: 7g
- Sugar: 8g

4. Dinner: Turkey and Vegetable Skewers with Brown Rice

Ingredients:

- 8 oz turkey breast, cut into cubes
- Mixed vegetables (bell peppers, cherry tomatoes, red onion)
- 1 cup brown rice (cooked)

Instructions:

- Skewer turkey and a variety of vegetables, grill, and serve with brown rice.

Nutritional Information:

- Calories: 380
- Protein: 30g
- Sugar: 3g

Cooking Time: 20 minutes

DAY 23 (TEUSDAY)

1. Breakfast: Spinach and Mushroom Omelette with Whole Wheat Toast

Ingredients:

- 3 large eggs
- Handful of fresh spinach
- 1/2 cup sliced mushrooms
- 2 slices whole wheat bread

Instructions:

1. Whisk eggs, sauté spinach and mushrooms, and pour over eggs.
2. Serve with whole wheat toast.

Nutritional Information:

- Calories: 350
- Protein: 20g
- Sugar: 3g

Cooking Time: 15 minutes

2. Lunch: Quinoa and Black Bean Bowl with Avocado

Ingredients:

- 1 cup quinoa (cooked)
- 1/2 cup black beans (canned, rinsed)
- Corn kernels
- 1/2 avocado, sliced

Instructions:

1. Combine quinoa, black beans, corn, and top with sliced avocado.

Nutritional Information:

- Calories: 380
- Protein: 15g

- Sugar: 5g

3. Snack: Cottage Cheese with Pineapple Chunks

Ingredients:

- 1/2 cup low-fat cottage cheese
- 1/2 cup pineapple chunks

Nutritional Information:

- Calories: 150
- Protein: 12g
- Sugar: 8g

4. Dinner: Baked Chicken Thighs with Sweet Potato Mash

Ingredients:

- 6 oz chicken thighs
- 1 medium sweet potato, mashed

Instructions:

2. Bake chicken thighs, serve with mashed sweet potatoes.

Nutritional Information:

- Calories: 450
- Protein: 30g
- Sugar: 6g

Cooking Time: 35 minutes

DAY 24 (WEDNESDAY)

1. Breakfast: Chia Seed Pudding Parfait with Mixed Berries

Ingredients:

- 2 tbsp chia seeds
- 1 cup unsweetened almond milk
- 1/2 cup mixed berries
- 1/4 cup Greek yogurt

Instructions:

1. Layer chia seed pudding with mixed berries and a dollop of Greek yogurt.

Nutritional Information:

- Calories: 250
- Protein: 7g
- Sugar: 6g

Preparation Time: 5 minutes (plus overnight refrigeration)

2. Lunch: Caprese Salad with Grilled Shrimp

Ingredients:

- 8 oz grilled shrimp
- Tomato slices
- Fresh mozzarella slices
- Fresh basil leaves
- Balsamic glaze

Instructions:

1. Combine tomato slices, fresh mozzarella, basil, and grilled shrimp.
2. Drizzle with balsamic glaze.

Nutritional Information:

- Calories: 350
- Protein: 25g
- Sugar: 5g

3. Snack: Greek Yogurt with Berries and Granola

Ingredients:

- 1 cup plain Greek yogurt
- 1/2 cup mixed berries (strawberries, blueberries)
- 2 tbsp granola

Nutritional Information:

- Calories: 250
- Protein: 15g
- Sugar: 10g

4. Dinner: Teriyaki Salmon with Stir-Fried Vegetables and Brown Rice

Ingredients:

- 6 oz salmon fillet
- Teriyaki sauce
- Mixed stir-fried vegetables (broccoli, snap peas, carrots)
- 1 cup brown rice (cooked)

Nutritional Information:

- Calories: 420
- Protein: 30g
- Sugar: 5g

Cooking Time: 25 minutes

DAY 25 (THURSDAY)

1. Breakfast: Banana Walnut Protein Pancakes

Ingredients:

- Whole wheat pancake mix
- 1 ripe banana, mashed
- Handful of chopped walnuts

Instructions:

- Mix whole wheat pancake batter with mashed bananas and chopped walnuts.
- Cook on a griddle.

Nutritional Information:

- Calories: 350
- Protein: 15g
- Sugar: 8g

Cooking Time: 15 minutes

2. Lunch: Turkey and Veggie Wrap with Hummus

Ingredients:

- 4 oz sliced turkey breast
- Whole wheat tortilla
- Mixed veggies (bell peppers, cucumber, lettuce)
- 2 tbsp hummus

Instructions:

1. Fill a whole wheat wrap with sliced turkey, assorted veggies, and a generous spread of hummus.

Nutritional Information:

- Calories: 380
- Protein: 20g
- Sugar: 4g

3. Snack: Mango and Cottage Cheese Parfait

Ingredients:

- 1/2 cup low-fat cottage cheese
- 1 ripe mango, diced
- 2 tbsp granola

Nutritional Information:

- Calories: 200
- Protein: 12g
- Sugar: 14g

4. Dinner: Grilled Chicken Salad with Quinoa

Ingredients:

- 6 oz grilled chicken breast
- Mixed greens
- 1/2 cup cherry tomatoes, halved
- 1/2 cup quinoa (cooked)
- Balsamic vinaigrette for dressing

Instructions:

- Grill chicken, place it on a bed of mixed greens, cherry tomatoes, and quinoa.
- Drizzle with balsamic vinaigrette.

Nutritional Information:

- Calories: 420
- Protein: 30g
- Sugar: 5g

Cooking Time: 25 minutes

DAY 26 (FRIDAY)

1. Breakfast: Spinach and Feta Egg Muffins

Ingredients:

- 3 large eggs
- Handful of fresh spinach, sautéed
- 2 tbsp crumbled feta cheese

Instructions:

1. Whisk eggs, mix with sautéed spinach and feta,
2. Pour into muffin tins, and bake.

Nutritional Information:

- Calories: 250
- Protein: 15g
- Sugar: 2g

Cooking Time: 20 minutes

2. Lunch: Quinoa and Black Bean Stuffed Bell Peppers

Ingredients:

- 1 cup quinoa (cooked)
- 1/2 cup black beans (canned, rinsed)
- Corn kernels
- 2 bell peppers, halved

Instructions:

1. Mix cooked quinoa with black beans, corn, and stuff into bell peppers.

2. Bake until peppers are tender.

Nutritional Information:

- Calories: 350
- Protein: 18g
- Sugar: 5g

Cooking Time: 30 minutes

3. Snack: Greek Yogurt with Pineapple and Almonds

Ingredients:

- 1 cup plain Greek yogurt
- 1/2 cup pineapple chunks
- 2 tbsp sliced almonds

Nutritional Information:

- Calories: 250
- Protein: 15g
- Sugar: 8g

4. Dinner: Baked Cod with Lemon and Dill

Ingredients:

- 6 oz cod fillet
- Lemon slices
- Fresh dill
- 1 cup steamed broccoli
- 1/2 cup quinoa (cooked)

Instructions:

1. Season cod with lemon and dill, bake until flaky.
2. Serve with steamed broccoli and quinoa.

Nutritional Information:

- Calories: 400
- Protein: 30g
- Sugar: 3g

Cooking Time: 25 minutes

DAY 27 (SATURDAY)

1. Breakfast: Almond Butter and Banana Smoothie

Ingredients:

- 2 tbsp almond butter
- 1 banana
- 1/2 cup Greek yogurt
- 1 cup unsweetened almond milk

Instructions:
1. Blend almond butter, banana, Greek yogurt, and almond milk until smooth.

Nutritional Information:
- Calories: 300
- Protein: 10g
- Sugar: 10g

2. *Lunch: Chickpea and Spinach Salad with Tahini Dressing*

Ingredients:
- 1 cup canned chickpeas (rinsed)
- Handful of fresh spinach
- 1/2 cup cherry tomatoes, halved
- 1/2 cucumber, diced
- Tahini dressing

Instructions:
1. Toss chickpeas, fresh spinach, cherry tomatoes, and cucumber.
2. Drizzle with tahini dressing

Nutritional Information:
- Calories: 320
- Protein: 14g
- Sugar: 6g

3. *Snack: Whole Grain Crackers with Hummus*

Ingredients:
- 1 serving whole grain crackers
- 4 tbsp hummus

Nutritional Information:
- Calories: 200
- Protein: 5g
- Sugar: 2g

4. *Dinner: Vegetable Stir-Fry with Tofu and Brown Rice*

Ingredients:
- 8 oz tofu, cubed
- Mixed vegetables (broccoli, bell peppers, snap peas)
- 1 cup brown rice (cooked)
- Soy sauce for seasoning

Instructions:
1. Stir-fry tofu and a mix of colorful vegetables in soy sauce.
2. Serve over brown rice.

Nutritional Information:

- Calories: 380
- Protein: 20g
- Sugar: 2g

Cooking Time: 20 minutes

DAY 28 (SUNDAY)

1. Breakfast Overnight Chia Seed Pudding with Mixed Berries

Ingredients:

- 2 tbsp chia seeds
- 1 cup unsweetened almond milk
- 1 tbsp honey
- 1/2 cup mixed berries

Instructions:

- Mix chia seeds, almond milk, and a touch of honey.
- Refrigerate overnight, and top with mixed berries.

Nutritional Information:

- Calories: 250
- Protein: 7g
- Sugar: 10g

Preparation Time: 5 minutes (plus overnight refrigeration)

2. Lunch: Mediterranean Chicken Wrap

Ingredients:

- 6 oz grilled chicken breast
- Whole wheat tortilla
- 2 tbsp hummus
- Cherry tomatoes, halved
- 1/2 cucumber, sliced
- 2 tbsp crumbled feta cheese

Instructions:

1. Fill a whole wheat wrap with grilled chicken, hummus, cherry tomatoes, cucumber, and feta cheese.

Nutritional Information:

- Calories: 380
- Protein: 25g
- Sugar: 4g

3. Snack: Edamame and Red Pepper Slices

Ingredients:

- 1 cup edamame (boiled)
- 1 red bell pepper, sliced

Nutritional Information:

- Calories: 150
- Protein: 12g
- Sugar: 6g

4. Dinner: Lentil and Vegetable Curry with Quinoa

Ingredients:

- 1 cup cooked lentils
- Mixed vegetables (cauliflower, carrots, peas)
- Curry sauce
- 1 cup quinoa (cooked)

Instructions:

1. Prepare a flavorful lentil and vegetable curry, serve over quinoa.

Nutritional Information:

- Calories: 400
- Protein: 18g
- Sugar: 5g

Cooking Time: 30 minutes

DAY 30

1. Breakfast: Smoked Salmon and Avocado Bagel

Ingredients:

- 1 whole grain bagel, toasted
- 2 oz smoked salmon
- 1/2 avocado, sliced
- Cream cheese for spreading
- Capers for garnish

Instructions:

1. Toast a whole grain bagel, spread cream cheese, and top with smoked salmon, avocado, and capers.

Nutritional Information:

- Calories: 350
- Protein: 20g
- Sugar: 3g

2. Lunch: Quinoa Bowl with Roasted Vegetables and Tahini Dressing

Ingredients:

- 1 cup quinoa (cooked)
- Mixed roasted vegetables (sweet potatoes, bell peppers, zucchini)
- Tahini dressing

Instructions:

1. Roast a variety of vegetables, serve over quinoa, and drizzle with tahini dressing.

Nutritional Information:

- Calories: 400
- Protein: 15g
- Sugar: 6g

Cooking Time: 25 minutes

3. Snack: Greek Yogurt and Berry Smoothie

Ingredients:

- 1 cup plain Greek yogurt
- 1/2 cup mixed berries (strawberries, blueberries)
- 1/4 cup granola

Nutritional Information:

- Calories: 250
- Protein: 15g
- Sugar: 8g

4. Dinner: Baked Falafel with Tzatziki Sauce and Pita Bread

Ingredients:

- Baked falafel (store-bought or homemade)
- Tzatziki sauce
- Whole wheat pita bread

Instructions:

1. Bake falafel, serve with tzatziki sauce, and whole wheat pita bread.

Nutritional Information:

- Calories: 380
- Protein: 18g
- Sugar: 4g

Cooking Time: 30 minutes

SNACKS AND SWEETS (THROUGHOUT THE MONTH)

1. Dark Chocolate-Dipped Strawberries

Ingredients:

- Fresh strawberries (150g / 5.3 oz)
- Dark chocolate (70% cocoa or higher) (50g / 1.8 oz)

Instructions:

1. Use a heat-resistant basin to melt dark chocolate.
2. Submerge each strawberry in the chocolate that has melted.
3. After putting it on parchment paper, allow it to cool until the chocolate solidifies.

Nutritional Information (per serving):

- Calories: 100 kcal
- Protein: 1g
- Sugars: 10g

Preparation Time: 15 minutes (excluding cooling time)

2. Chia Seed Pudding with Berries

Ingredients:

- Almond milk (unsweetened) (200ml / 6.8 fl oz)
- Chia seeds (30g / 1 oz)
- Mixed berries (strawberries, blueberries) (100g / 3.5 oz)
- Honey or sweetener (optional)

Instructions:

1. Combine almond milk and chia seeds, then refrigerate for the entire night.
2. Arrange mixed berries on top of chia pudding in the morning.
3. If preferred, sweeten with honey or another sweetener.

Nutritional Information (per serving):

- Calories: 200 kcal
- Protein: 5g
- Sugars: 5g

Preparation Time: Overnight (plus 10 minutes in the morning)

3. Trail Mix with Dried Fruits and Nuts

Ingredients:

- Dark chocolate chips (optional) (15g / 0.5 oz)
- Dried fruits (raisins, cranberries) (30g / 1 oz)
- Mixed nuts (almonds, walnuts, pistachios) (30g / 1 oz)

Instructions:

1. Add the dark chocolate chips, mixed nuts, and dried fruits together.
2. Divide into portions the size of snacks.

Nutritional Information (per serving):

- Calories: 150 kcal
- Protein: 3g
- Sugars: 8g

Preparation Time: 5 minutes

4. Baked Apple with Cinnamon

Ingredients:

- Cinnamon
- Apple (1 medium)
- Honey or sweetener (optional)

Instructions:

1. Cut the apple into cores and dust with cinnamon.
2. Bake until the apple becomes soft.
3. Drizzle with honey or sugar, if preferred.

Nutritional Information (per serving):

- Calories: 80 kcal
- Protein: 1g
- Sugars: 15g

Preparation Time: 20 minutes

5. Avocado and Tomato Salsa

Ingredients:

- Lime juice (1 tablespoon)
- Avocado (1 medium, diced)
- Tomatoes (2 medium, diced)
- Fresh cilantro (chopped)
- Red onion (1/4 cup, finely chopped)

Instructions:

1. In a bowl, mix chopped avocado, tomatoes, red onion, cilantro, and lime juice.
2. Combine thoroughly and serve with veggie sticks or whole-grain crackers.

Nutritional Information (per serving):

- Calories: 120 kcal
- Protein: 2g
- Sugars: 3g

Preparation Time: 10 minutes

6. Cauliflower Rice Stir-Fry with Chicken

Ingredients:

- Cauliflower rice (150g / 5.3 oz)
- Chicken breast (cooked and shredded) (100g / 3.5 oz)
- Mixed vegetables (bell peppers, broccoli) (100g / 3.5 oz)
- Soy sauce (low-sodium)
- Sesame oil

Instructions:

1. Combine mixed veggies, shredded chicken, and cauliflower rice in a sesame oil stir-fry.
2. For taste, add soy sauce.

Nutritional Information (per serving):

- Calories: 150 kcal
- Protein: 15g
- Sugars: 5g

Preparation Time: 15 minutes

7. Yogurt-Covered Blueberries

Ingredients:

- Blueberries (100g / 3.5 oz)
- Greek yogurt (unsweetened) (100g / 3.5 oz)

Instructions:

1. Until coated, dip each blueberry into the Greek yogurt.
2. Transfer to a dish lined with parchment paper, then freeze until the yogurt solidifies.

Nutritional Information (per serving):

- Calories: 50 kcal
- Protein: 3g
- Sugars: 5g

Preparation Time: 10 minutes (plus freezing time)

8. Ricotta and Berry Parfait

Ingredients:

- Mixed berries (strawberries, blueberries) (100g / 3.5 oz)
- Ricotta cheese (150g / 5.3 oz)
- Honey or sweetener (optional)

Instructions:

- Arrange a layer of mixed berries and ricotta cheese in a glass.
- Use honey or another sweetener, if preferred.

Nutritional Information (per serving):

- Calories: 180 kcal

- Protein: 10g
- Sugars: 8g

Preparation Time: 5 minutes

9. Baked Pear with Cinnamon and Walnuts

Ingredients:

- Walnuts (crushed) (15g / 0.5 oz)
- Pear (1 medium, sliced)
- Cinnamon
- Honey or sweetener (optional)

Instructions:

1. Arrange the pear slices and dust them with cinnamon on a baking sheet.
2. Bake the pear until it is soft.
3. Sprinkle chopped walnuts on top and, if preferred, drizzle with honey or another sweetness.

Nutritional Information (per serving):

- Calories: 120 kcal
- Protein: 2g
- Sugars: 15g

Preparation Time: 20 minutes

10. Coconut and Almond Energy Bites

Ingredients:

- Shredded coconut (30g / 1 oz)
- Almond flour (50g / 1.8 oz)
- Vanilla extract (1/2 teaspoon)
- Almond butter (unsweetened) (2 tablespoons)
- Honey (1 tablespoon)

Instructions:

1. In a bowl, combine almond flour, honey, vanilla essence, shredded coconut, and almond butter.
2. Form into little balls and chill until solid.

Nutritional Information (per serving):

- Calories: 120 kcal
- Protein: 4g
- Sugars: 5g

Preparation Time: 15 minutes (plus refrigeration time)

11. Caprese Skewers

Ingredients:

- Fresh mozzarella balls (bocconcini) (150g / 5.3 oz)

- Cherry tomatoes (200g / 7 oz)
- Balsamic glaze
- Olive oil (extra virgin)
- Fresh basil leaves
- Salt and pepper to taste

Instructions:

1. Thread a cherry tomato, a mozzarella ball, and a leaf of fresh basil onto each skewer.
2. Put the skewers in order on a dish for serving.
3. Drizzle olive oil and balsamic glaze over.
4. Add salt and pepper to taste.

Nutritional Information (per serving):

- Calories: 100 kcal
- Protein: 5g
- Sugars: 2g

Preparation Time: 15 minutes

12. Cabbage Rolls with Lean Beef and Brown Rice

Ingredients:

- Brown rice (cooked) (1 cup)
- Cabbage leaves (8 large)
- Lean ground beef (250g / 8.8 oz)
- Tomato sauce (low-sugar) (400ml / 13.5 fl oz)
- Onion (1 medium, finely chopped)
- Italian seasoning
- Garlic (minced)
- Salt and pepper to taste

Instructions:

1. Simmer cabbage leaves till tender, then remove and set aside.
2. Combine cooked brown rice, Italian seasoning, onion, and garlic with ground meat in a bowl.
3. Roll each cabbage leaf with a spoonful of the beef mixture.
4. Spread the rolls out in a baking dish, pour tomato sauce over them, and bake for about 30 minutes or until done.

Nutritional Information (per serving):

- Calories: 250 kcal
- Protein: 15g
- Sugars: 5g

Preparation Time: 45 minutes

13. Pumpkin Seed Trail Mix

Ingredients:

- Almonds (30g / 1 oz)

- Pumpkin seeds (pepitas) (100g / 3.5 oz)
- Dark chocolate chips (optional) (30g / 1 oz)
- Dried cranberries (30g / 1 oz)

Instructions:

1. Mix dark chocolate chips, almonds, dried cranberries, and pumpkin seeds.
2. Thoroughly combine and divide into snack-sized portions.

Nutritional Information (per serving):

- Calories: 150 kcal
- Protein: 5g
- Sugars: 5g

Preparation Time: 10 minutes

14. Cherry Almond Biscotti

Ingredients:

- Almonds (50g / 1.8 oz, chopped)
- Almond flour (150g / 5.3 oz)
- Almond extract (1 teaspoon)
- Dried cherries (50g / 1.8 oz)
- Honey (3 tablespoons)
- Eggs (2 large)
- Baking powder (1 teaspoon)

Instructions:

1. Set a baking sheet covered with parchment paper and preheat the oven.
2. Combine almond flour, eggs, honey, almond extract, sliced almonds, dried cherries, and baking powder in a bowl.
3. On the baking sheet, form the dough into a log and bake it until it becomes hard.
4. Cut the log into biscotti shapes, then re-bake it until it turns brown.

Nutritional Information (per serving):

- Calories: 120 kcal
- Protein: 4g
- Sugars: 8g

Preparation Time: 30 minutes

15. Apricot and Walnut Oat Bars

Ingredients:

- Dried apricots (100g / 3.5 oz, chopped)
- Rolled oats (200g / 7 oz)
- Honey (3 tablespoons)
- Walnuts (50g / 1.8 oz, chopped)
- Vanilla extract (1 teaspoon)
- Almond butter (100g / 3.5 oz)

Instructions:
1. Preheat the oven and place parchment paper inside a baking dish.
2. Combine the rolled oats, almond butter, honey, chopped walnuts, dried apricots, and vanilla extract in a bowl.
3. Transfer the mixture to the baking dish and bake it for a golden color
4. Let it cool before slicing it into bars.

Nutritional Information (per serving):
- Calories: 180 kcal
- Protein: 5g
- Sugars: 10g

Preparation Time: 25 minutes

16. Baked Banana with Cinnamon and Walnuts

Ingredients:
- Walnuts (15g / 0.5 oz, chopped)
- Cinnamon
- Banana (1 medium, sliced)
- Honey or sweetener (optional)

Instructions:
1. Arrange the slices of banana on a baking pan.
2. Add chopped walnuts and cinnamon to the mixture.
3. Bake the banana until it's tender.
4. If preferred, drizzle with honey or another sweetness.

Nutritional Information (per serving):
- Calories: 150 kcal
- Protein: 3g
- Sugars: 10g

Preparation Time: 15 minutes

17. Cinnamon Roasted Walnuts

Ingredients:
- Maple syrup (1 tablespoon)
- Cinnamon
- Walnuts (150g / 5.3 oz)
- Sea salt to taste

Instructions:
1. Set a baking sheet covered with parchment paper and preheat the oven.
2. Combine walnuts with maple syrup and cinnamon.
3. Transfer to a baking pan, scatter sea salt on top, and roast until aromatic.

Nutritional Information (per serving):
- Calories: 200 kcal
- Protein: 5g

- Sugars: 2g

Preparation Time: 20 minutes

18. Mediterranean Chickpea Salad

Ingredients:

- Cherry tomatoes (150g / 5.3 oz, halved)
- Chickpeas (canned, drained) (200g / 7 oz)
- Kalamata olives (50g / 1.8 oz, sliced)
- Cucumber (1 medium, diced)
- Red onion (1/4 cup, finely chopped)
- Feta cheese (50g / 1.8 oz, crumbled)
- Fresh parsley (chopped)
- Olive oil (extra virgin)
- Lemon juice
- Salt and pepper to taste

Instructions:

1. Put the cucumber, feta cheese, cherry tomatoes, olives, red onion, and chickpeas in a bowl.
2. Add a lemon juice and olive oil drizzle.
3. Include the fresh parsley and season with pepper and salt.

Nutritional Information (per serving):

- Calories: 250 kcal
- Protein: 10g
- Sugars: 3g

Preparation Time: 15 minutes

19. Frozen Grapes

Ingredients:

- Grapes (150g / 5.3 oz)

Instructions:

1. Wash and thoroughly dry the grapes.
2. Store in the freezer until solid.
3. Savour as a delicious and reviving frozen snack

Nutritional Information (per serving):

- Calories: 50 kcal
- Protein: 0.5g
- Sugars: 12g

Preparation Time: 2 hours (freezing time)

20. Homemade Guacamole with Veggie Sticks

Ingredients:

- Red onion (1/4 cup, finely chopped)
- Avocado (1 medium, mashed)
- Tomato (1 medium, diced)
- Lime juice
- Garlic (1 clove, minced)
- Carrot and cucumber sticks (for dipping)
- Fresh cilantro (chopped)

Instructions:

1. Combine mashed avocado, lime juice, fresh cilantro, diced tomato, red onion, and minced garlic in a bowl.
2. Gently stir, then serve with cucumber and carrot sticks.

Nutritional Information (per serving):

- Calories: 120 kcal
- Protein: 2g
- Sugars: 2g

Preparation Time: 10 minutes

21. Blueberry and Almond Baked Oatmeal Cups

Ingredients:

- Blueberries (100g / 3.5 oz)
- Rolled oats (1 cup)
- Almond milk (unsweetened) (240ml / 8 fl oz)
- Maple syrup (2 tablespoons)
- Almonds (30g / 1 oz, chopped)
- Vanilla extract (1 teaspoon)
- Egg (1 large)

Instructions:

1. Fit cupcake liners into a muffin tin and preheat the oven.
2. Combine the rolled oats, egg, vanilla extract, maple syrup, chopped almonds, blueberries, and almond milk in a bowl.
3. Spoon mixture into muffin tins; bake until firm.

Nutritional Information (per serving):

- Calories: 150 kcal
- Protein: 5g
- Sugars: 8g

Preparation Time: 25 minutes

22. Peach and Raspberry Yogurt Parfait

Ingredients:

- Greek yogurt (unsweetened) (200g / 7 oz)
- Peaches (1 medium, sliced)
- Granola (30g / 1 oz)
- Raspberries (100g / 3.5 oz)
- Honey or sweetener (optional)

Instructions:

Arrange Greek, granola, Ving):

- Calories: 250 kcal
- Protein: 10g
- Sugars: 12g

Preparation Time: 10 minutes

23. Greek Yogurt with Walnuts and Honey

Ingredients:

- Walnuts (20g / 0.7 oz, chopped)
- Greek yogurt (unsweetened) (150g / 5.3 oz)
- Honey or sweetener (optional)

Instructions:

1. Put chopped walnuts and Greek yogurt in a bowl.
2. If preferred, sweeten with honey or another sweetener.

Nutritional Information (per serving):

- Calories: 200 kcal
- Protein: 10g
- Sugars: 5g

Preparation Time: 5 minutes

24. Cauliflower and Broccoli Gratin

Ingredients:

- Butter (2 tablespoons)
- Broccoli (200g / 7 oz, florets)
- Milk (300ml / 10 fl oz)
- Cauliflower (200g / 7 oz, florets)
- All-purpose flour (2 tablespoons)
- Parmesan cheese (50g / 1.8 oz, grated)
- Cheddar cheese (100g / 3.5 oz, shredded)
- Nutmeg (1/4 teaspoon, grated)
- Garlic (2 cloves, minced)

- Salt and pepper to taste
- Breadcrumbs (optional, for topping)

Instructions:

1. Grease a baking dish and preheat the oven.
2. Boil or steam broccoli and cauliflower until just soft. Put them inside the dish for baking.
3. Melt butter in a pot over a medium heat. To make a roux, add the flour and whisk.
4. Add milk gradually while whisking until thickened and smooth.
5. Stir in the melted Parmesan and cheddar cheeses.
6. Season the cheese sauce with salt, pepper, nutmeg, and minced garlic. Drizzle the broccoli and cauliflower over top.
7. For an optional crunchy crust, top with breadcrumbs.
8. Bake till bubbling and golden brown on top.

Nutritional Information (per serving):

- Calories: 250 kcal
- Protein: 12g
- Sugars: 5g

Preparation Time: 40 minutes

25. Orange and Almond Muffins

Ingredients:

- Orange zest (2 tablespoons)
- Eggs (2 large)
- Almonds (50g / 1.8 oz, chopped)
- Almond flour (150g / 5.3 oz)
- Vanilla extract (1 teaspoon)
- Honey (3 tablespoons)
- Salt (1/4 teaspoon)
- Baking powder (1 teaspoon)

Instructions:

1. To make cake liners, preheat the oven and line a muffin tray.
2. 2 Almonds, eggs, honey, baking powder, vanilla essence, orange zest, chopped almonds, and salt should all be combined in a bowl.
3. After thoroughly mixing, ladle the batter into the muffin tins.
4. When a toothpick inserted into the muffins comes out clean, they are done baking.

Nutritional Information (per serving):

- Calories: 180 kcal
- Protein: 6g
- Sugars: 8g

Preparation Time: 25 minutes

26. Chocolate Avocado Mousse

Ingredients:

- Maple syrup (4 tablespoons)
- Cocoa powder (4 tablespoons)
- Avocado (2 ripe)
- Almond milk (unsweetened) (60ml / 2 fl oz)
- Vanilla extract (1 teaspoon)

Instructions:

1. Put the avocados (peeled and pitted), almond milk, chocolate powder, maple syrup, and vanilla extract in a blender.
2. Blend until creamy and smooth.
3. Let it cool in the fridge for a minimum of two hours prior to serving.

Nutritional Information (per serving):

- Calories: 200 kcal
- Protein: 3g
- Sugars: 15g

Preparation Time: 10 minutes + chilling time

27. Mixed Berry Sorbet

Ingredients:

- Water (60ml / 2 fl oz)
- Lemon juice (2 tablespoons)
- Mixed berries (strawberries, blueberries, raspberries) (300g / 10.6 oz)
- Honey or agave syrup (2 tablespoons)

Instructions:

1. Put water, lemon juice, agave syrup or honey, and mixed berries in a blender.
2. Blend until smooth.
3. Transfer the mixture to a shallow dish and place in the freezer.
4. Use a fork to stir the mixture once every hour until it takes on the consistency of sorbet.

Nutritional Information (per serving):

- Calories: 100 kcal
- Protein: 1g
- Sugars: 20g

Preparation Time: 10 minutes + freezing time

28. Pistachio and Cranberry Granola Bars

Ingredients:

- Pistachios (50g / 1.8 oz, chopped)
- Rolled oats (200g / 7 oz)
- Honey (4 tablespoons)
- Dried cranberries (50g / 1.8 oz)

- Vanilla extract (1 teaspoon)
- Almond butter (4 tablespoons)
- Salt (1/4 teaspoon)

Instructions:

1. Preheat the oven and place parchment paper inside a baking dish.
2. Combine rolled oats, chopped almonds, dried cranberries, honey, almond butter, vanilla essence, and salt in a bowl.
3. Transfer the mixture to the baking dish and bake it for a golden color.
4. Let cool completely before slicing into bars of granola.

Nutritional Information (per serving):

- Calories: 200 kcal
- Protein: 5g
- Sugars: 15g

Preparation Time: 15 minutes + cooling time

Don't forget to scan the
QR Code to get all bonus content!

Printed in Great Britain
by Amazon

36143933R00071